*A Story of UnPlanned Parenthood
and the Case for Life*

Choose
Zoe

BY LAURA LYNN HUGHES

ENDORSEMENTS

"An unplanned pregnancy, like so many situations in life, can throw us for a loop and lead us into hopelessness and despair. But with great wisdom, insight, and vulnerability, Laura Lynn Hughes shares her own moving testimony and reminds us that we serve a God who anoints every single human life with great value, hope, and potential."

Jim Daly, President of *Focus on the Family*

"An amazing journey from teenage victim to life champion."

Jor-El Godsey, President of *Heartbeat Internationalily*

"The prolife movement does not point fingers of condemnation at the world, but rather extends hands of mercy, hope, and strength. Choose Zoe demonstrates that powerfully, and I urge you to absorb its message and pass it on."

Fr. Frank Pavone, National Director of *Priests for Life*; Pastoral Director of *Rachel's Vineyard* and *Silent No More*

"Laura has poured out her heart and unleashed the argument of love. Her vulnerable words are passionate, powerful and wholly inspirational."

Carey Wickersham, Author of *The Wonder Within You*

CONTENTS

 Download the free Live Portrait app on your Android or iPhone and scan the special photos in this book identified with the Live Portrait Logo to see the embedded video.

A Note on My Title

Some people have asked, when hearing the title of my book, if my daughter's name is Zoe. While that would be terribly convenient, it is not the case. And, unfortunately, after living for forty years with a different name, she doesn't seem inclined to change it now.

No, the title of my book comes from my love of the Greek language, and how using it while studying Scripture has helped me understand God and the transformative power of His Word. I love how a word that we take for granted to mean one thing in English can have multiple meanings in the original biblical languages.

Life is one such word. In Greek, *life* is translated as physical life, or *bios*; psychological life, or *psuche*; and finally, abundant, divine life: *zoe*. God knew that life based solely on the physical and psychological could be painful, delicate, sometimes cut short, and something we shouldn't take for granted. It would be challenging, heartbreaking, tragic, and at times unfair. That is why Jesus offers us so much more:

zoe—the eternal, divine, abundant life. His original design was for humanity to live with a fullness of abundant life in communion with Him, and it is this final description of life that has captured my heart.

Used 127 times in the New Testament, *zoe* is a constant reminder of the fullness that God intended for His people. In John 10:10, Jesus says, "I have come that they may have *zoe* and have *zoe* more abundantly." Jesus repeatedly offers this to us, whether to the woman at the well in John 4:14 or the five thousand who are fed in John 6:35. Our Bible begins with *zoe*, when God places the Tree of Life *(Zoe)* in the Garden of Eden in Genesis 2, and it ends with it as well. In Revelation 22 we are told that, because of Christ's sacrifice, we again have access to the Tree of *Zoe*.

Since the most important book in my world begins with *zoe*, I thought it would be a good place to start mine.

CHAPTER 1

Beginnings

It was thirty-nine years ago, but I remember like it was yesterday. I was fifteen years old and looking out the picture window of our kitchen. The early spring sun lit up a world slowly waking from winter, bringing forth new life. Smells of Mom's Easter feast were wafting from the kitchen. In the front yard, my sister-in-law and two of my sisters were lined up sideways, showing off their baby bumps. My dad, the proud grandfather-to-be, stood ready with his camera.

"Okay, smile, all my pregnant girls!"

I felt a kick. A sweet little baby kick. Only I knew that I belonged in the picture too. I wanted to be out there, the breeze stirring my plaid smock with cherries on the pockets around my baby bump as I turned sideways and made known the beginnings of a new life within me. How had it gone undetected this long? What would my family do when they found out? My family was Irish, and keeping true to our religious heritage, we were Roman Catholic. Would the shame of my situation rule out my place in the image? I put my hands on my belly to better feel the movement. Though my heart was racing, I felt peaceful inside. Nothing, not even the unpredictable reaction from my parents, could overshadow hope and the budding love for my unborn child.

Some beginnings are hard. As a little girl, I would have argued to the contrary. Surrounded by adoring parents and seven older siblings, I knew very little about difficulty. Growing up under the wide-open Montana sky, my joy knew no bounds. Never had a child been as loved and adored. My memories are full of images of dancing on tables, being carted around on my older brothers' shoulders, being read to and doted on incessantly.

It wasn't that my family did not have struggles or pain; it was simply that my happiness was oblivious to sorrow. After my birth, Mom suffered a miscarriage. She couldn't stop bleeding for weeks and required a D&C.[i]

Since Dad traveled two weeks at a time for work, my eldest brother, Michael, had charge over my crib and nighttime feedings. Mom grew more and more worn out, and Dad needed a lot of help with us. When I was two, my mother was hospitalized with rheumatic fever for seven months, and the doctor declared she needed bed rest for several more months. As the two youngest, my brother Joe—older by two years—and I were sent five hours away to Augusta, Montana, to live with my grandparents. They were respected in the

---

i   A D&C stands for dilation and curettage. A doctor opens the cervix and surgically remove the contents of the uterus by scraping the uterine wall with a sharp tool, called a curette, or by suction. D&C's are used when women have lost a baby but are having difficulty passing the remains. They are also the tool of choice for late-term abortion doctors. Except, in their case, they use the curette to dissect the live baby into smaller parts so that it can be more easily suctioned out of the body.

small rural town: My grandmother was renowned for being in the Cowboy Hall of Fame and the first female postmaster. Both she and my grandfather served as postmasters during the war, and our family owned the general store. Between the town's feelings for our grandparents and their pity for our situation, we were indulged by everyone. The postman brought us Black Jack gum; the milkman brought us Lemonheads; the staff at the general store always turned a blind eye to our pillaging of the penny candy. We lived with my grandparents for two years—jumping in their bed every morning to be gummed by my grandmother before she put in her dentures. Joe and I were the center of their world. I remember it as a sweet time, literally and figuratively. After we were reunited with our recovered mother and family, existence continued in its easy way for me.

I had always imagined life would carry on in pretty much the same fashion as my family. I would fall in love with a man who cherished me and treated me like my father treated my mother. We would marry, have a houseful of children like my parents had, and spend the rest of our days in bliss. Even as a small girl, I knew I wanted to be a mother. It was the dream that overshadowed all others. But the beginning of that dream's fruition was much different than I had planned. Little did I suspect that the moment at the window would give me vision for my life's work—to advocate for life.

From rape, incest, or sex-trafficking survivors, to the women who walk into the clinic where I volunteer, to those who, like my daughter, have chosen abortion, and finally to my own story, I have and always will "choose life." But before I get into those stories and explain how I ended up becoming an advocate for life, let me first describe what it actually means to me.

Life.

Such a small word for such a huge concept. Regardless of faith or religious background, everyone can agree on this: Life is awe-inspiring. It persists; whether it is as small as minute organisms on this earth or as complex as the humans who populate the planet, nature reproduces and survives. Life has its own, God-breathed energy, and it's unstoppable.

In the beginning, when the world was dark and formless, God's spirit hovered over the chaotic waters and brought order. He breathed *life!* He offered *zoe*—which means eternal, divine, abundant life—by planting the Tree of Life, or the Tree of "Zoe," in the Garden of Eden. But sadly, humanity wanted more and rejected the abundant life in favor of knowledge and power. We wanted choice, and God granted it. But for our arrogance and rebellion, we lost access to the Tree of Zoe and tried to fill our lives with poor substitutes for countless generations. Then...

Mercy.

Grace.

Redemption.

God sent His son, who took our arrogance and rebellion upon Himself and died for our transgressions. In exchange for our sin, He freely offered access to the Tree of Zoe once again. The example of Jesus shows us what a life of zoe is all about: having mercy and compassion, sacrificing for others, choosing hope in the face of despair, and an abundant life. It's a life that may not be void of trouble, but with which He will provide the grace to live well with peace and joy, believing we serve a good God who holds our futures in His hands.

Merely surviving is not enough.

How do I know? Because *I* am more than a survivor. At the age of ten, I encountered trauma at an unexpected place. My family frequented the pancake breakfasts held by a local charitable society. Where else could a family of ten eat for a dollar? We children were left to roam with our friends, and on this particular day I was playing in one of the empty banquet rooms with some older boys who were classmates of my brother, and one boy who was my friend. We chased each other around the many banquet tables, which were all spread with perfectly white tablecloths—a sea of white in an otherwise dark room.

At one point we gathered under the same table, and it was there, in that deserted room, under a shrouded banquet table, they molested me. Time stood still. I was frozen. My friend from my class didn't participate, but he just sat there and watched, not even trying to defend me. Even though I had no concept of sex at that age, I immediately felt worthless and dirty. When they were finished, they left me there. I lay there for a while before fumbling with my jeans clasp, but my fingers were numb, as was the rest of me.

When I walked out of that room and shut the door, I closed the door on the memory as well. I didn't directly think about it again for decades. But that night, the nightmares started. Horrible nightmares that usually involved me floating above a scene where someone I loved was being harmed, and I was powerless to do anything. I began wetting the bed and sleepwalking. My parents had to make sure the doors were secure at night or I would wander outside. The happy poetry I loved to write turned dark.

And no one asked why.

I was isolated in my pain. My ten-year-old brain couldn't process what had happened. I needed the loving guidance of a trusted adult, but my family didn't talk about such things. Raised in such innocence, I was unable to articulate the unthinkable. We were a good, loving, faithful Roman Catholic family that lived well religiously, but never delved into such intense topics.

Shame and self-loathing were introduced into my life the day the abuse occurred. Though I blocked the memory of the event for many years, the feelings remained. It became easier and easier to believe that I was worthless. I allowed those lies to live in the back of my mind, not knowing their origin. It wasn't until just recently that I had a powerful encounter with God that changed everything. The memory was made crystal clear to me, and in that moment with God, He took the tablecloth that had hidden the shameful act, and wrapped it around my shoulders instead, clothing me in righteousness. He reminded me that I am royalty—His child and masterpiece. I no longer needed to feel the shame or believe the lies. The truth was:

I didn't deserve the abuse...

It wasn't my fault...

I wasn't a bad person because it happened to me...

It wasn't my legacy, or the legacy of my children...

The abusive experience and its aftereffects have proven to be a very challenging part of my life. Yet even in the midst of the pain, shame, and subsequent choices born out of that situation, I did more than survive. How? God brought me to the Tree of Zoe, and I have experienced the life of abundance that results from showing mercy, living sacrificially, offering hope, and believing in a good God despite what happened to me.

But just like humanity in the beginning, each of us must decide between choosing a zoe life made available to us freely through Jesus's sacrifice or choosing to merely survive in this fallen world. Embracing this truth empowers each of us to create lives of peace, joy, and fulfillment that we all desire. Otherwise fear, lack, and hopelessness dictate our destiny.

When you hear the phrase "choose life," especially in today's political climate, it is often the *bios*, or physical life, that comes to mind. We want the unborn to be saved, and we also want to save lives from war, famine, devastation, and from sin. These are essential, and I will be examining the momentous decision to choose physical life for our unborn throughout the book. As noble as these desires and efforts are, however, I would argue that our calling, and what is truly needed to change the world, is to choose not just *bios*, but *zoe*. God has so much more for us than mere physical existence. We were created to thrive.

So, how do we actually *choose zoe*? Where do we begin? First, we must believe we are worthy of the abundant lives God has sacrificed for and called us to live—and not only in the material meaning that is often synonymous with *abundance*. Once we have grasped this truth for ourselves, we have to wholeheartedly believe God wants this for *everyone*, and that He wants to use *us* to make it a reality.

Further, we must know that because we are children of God, every single person has intrinsic, incalculable value, that the breath of God that gives all of us life is sacred. This belief in the sacredness of life—or in what has taken on an almost exclusively political connotation and lost meaning as of late, the *sanctity* of life—is an important part of establishing the framework in which a zoe life can flourish. This ethic upholds the creed that all human life is sacred and possesses inherent dignity and value by its sheer existence, regardless of circumstance. Modern culture promotes the idea that life is only worth living if it meets a certain standard (and who gets to decide that standard is anyone's guess). Thus, some argue that only a "good" life, in which certain financial or health standards are met, is a valuable one. But since there is no arbitrary measure of a "good" life in order to decide if someone should be given the opportunity to live, again, who decides? Honoring sanctity of life in no way nullifies quality of life, as we are called to make this world better for all. It does, however, reject the notion that a subjective standard should rule out life altogether.

Choosing the zoe life means that sanctity of life doesn't end at birth, because life isn't about simply existing. Sanctity of life is about dignity for all human life in all stages. That means caring for mothers after they give birth and for children born into difficult circumstances. It means advocating for the immigrant, the elderly, the disabled, and all those marginalized by society. And it means caring for and loving women who have chosen abortion. It implies treating all people with respect, regardless of their background, political standing, financial circumstances, religious beliefs, or even likeability. Without respect, there is no dignity, and we can't claim all life has dignity if we don't show it with our actions. God offers zoe equally to everyone. He has called us to reach for it and to help others do the same. We are not the keepers of zoe, or some sort of vessel deciding upon whom it gets dispensed. Rather, we are the conduit.

I can think of no better example of this than my own mother, Sally. She had so much of a zoe life that it spilled out onto everyone around her. She wasn't just a conduit; she was the Alaska pipeline. She worked hard raising eight kids and miraculously had dinner on the table every night by six o'clock sharp. Yet, somehow she managed to do a host of other things as well. Not only did she volunteer at our school, but she also donated her time to the hospital, pregnancy care center, prison, halfway house, and the Montana Mission. Despite all those endeavors, Mom always expressed that her main ministry was her family.

I get a little lightheaded thinking about accomplishing half of that. But accomplish it she did, and with a loving and pure heart. No one knew about several of these endeavors until her death, when former meth addicts and convicted felons began showing up to pay their respects. Former inmates of the women's prison even held a picnic in her honor and invited our family. The people she touched individually while quietly carrying out her zoe life could easily fill a book. When she was on her deathbed, the hospice chaplain came to visit with her. They were good friends because she volunteered with him frequently. When he left that day, he cried, telling me, "That is so like your mom. I came to bring her encouragement, and I'm the one who is leaving encouraged."

My mother was excited about life. We all know people who fall into one of two categories: those who live life to the fullest, taking advantage of every opportunity for adventure and exploration, and those who are, well, just trying not to die. Watch either for very long, and it will become clear who is getting the most out of life. In much the same way, creating a culture of life is about creating something positive, about offering people real choices that give them practical ways of living an abundant life. If the negative is always the focus, what is created is a culture of law that isn't life-giving. Church and faith become about keeping a list of rules and being motivated by fear and legalism, which brings about very little true heart change. Think about it: Would you rather have a child's actions inspired by love and the desire to do good, or by fear and avoidance of negative consequences? When faith becomes a culture of law, we lose the joy of choosing abundant life. Further, women and men who have not lived up to expectations hide in a prison of shame and judgment, afraid there is no room for them at the table of law and perfection.

Rather than spending all our energy on skirmishing with abortion-rights advocates, choosing a zoe life says that, as a society, we can do better than abortion. In a seemingly hopeless situation, there is a superior solution to ending a life. It isn't about screaming in picket lines or simply changing laws. First, we must change hearts. In democracy, the law will eventually catch up with the heart of the people. If hearts are changed, the law isn't needed—it will be written on our hearts.

How do we change people's hearts? We do it by offering hope. That is what people in crisis want. Hope is an essential ingredient to human life. When people lose it, they lose the will to live. Without God, unplanned pregnancy can have a hopeless end. With God, it can have endless hope.

Hurting people want options that give them a chance for life—real life, not just existence. They hope for zoe.

In 1 Corinthians 13:13 we are told that three things will remain: faith, hope, and love. All three are necessary for choosing zoe in difficult times. Hope drives our will to live; love drives that will on behalf of others; and faith gives assurance of a future with God. Women who are considering abortion need to feel hope that they can succeed and that there is a good plan for their lives. They need a love for their child that surpasses their own self-interest. Finally, they must have faith in the person helping them—God's representative in their situation.

Without God, unplanned pregnancy can have a hopeless end. With God, it can have endless hope.

Choosing zoe means we live wholeheartedly, facing pain and not allowing it to dictate our decisions or cause us to embrace addictions. It also means we make healthy emotional, physical, and spiritual life choices. We are called to embrace authentic and healthy living, not only for ourselves but for those around us. We must first implement these aspects of the zoe life so that we can, in turn, help others grasp it as well.

I would not presume to say that if a woman chooses life, her life will be picture perfect. No. Life is messy for all of us. Sometimes the chaos is the result of our own choices; sometimes it's the result of choices of those close to us. Either way, we can't escape debris. I would love to sit here and write, as I gaze with a sage look in my eye, that my life has turned out perfectly. I wish I could say that after choosing life for my baby, only goodness has come my way, that I have the dream: the 2.5 kids, the house with the white picket fence and the small yet family-sustainable garden in the backyard. Heck, maybe I even raise my own chickens—a girl can dream.

But that isn't reality. Reality is that I have had my continued share of struggles and heartache. I have had more than one failed marriage. I have single-parented five children, and at times they have made choices that hurt them and therefore me. And, if I may be glib, I stink at gardening. So why does someone like me—a flawed woman—feel the need to write a book about choosing zoe? Here's the thing: A decision I made at fifteen years of age created the framework for my life direction as an advocate.

I stand as an example of someone who did not always make the right choices, but who has been able to help moms, dads, rape victims, and those recovering from abortions and other trauma make the decision to choose life—a full life.

As you read on, you'll not only hear their stories, but also the rest of my own. You will read my thoughts on developing life-giving parent-child relationships, helping those who have unplanned pregnancies, choosing zoe in the midst of trauma and disability, the power of our image, the reality of abortion and how to heal from it, the pain of infertility and miscarriage, and the gift and sacrifice of adoption.

I have received uncountable blessings from what I consider to be my life's work, not only from those I have helped, but also from my children and grandchildren. And it was worth it all: the pain, the suffering, the sacrifice, the financial lack at times, and even the condemnation and judgment by others. The purpose of this book is to help people choose *zoe*, to choose *life*, not to heap criticism or shame on a single soul. I would be heartbroken if that is what someone took away from my story.

I stand as an example of someone who did not always make the right choices, but who has been able to help moms, dads, rape victims, and those recovering from abortions and other trauma make the decision to choose life—a full life.

God sees my deficiencies, and as He did in the beginning of time, His spirit hovers over the chaos in my life, bringing grace and offering zoe. Obviously, the result is not perfection. The result is an imperfect woman, desperately clinging to the Tree of Zoe, which God lovingly planted in her bedraggled backyard. The surrounding grass is uneven, and weeds ever sneak closer, trying in vain to climb its trunk. But the tree stands, immune to my failings. It isn't my tree. It's

God's. I choose whether or not to be in its presence, but nothing I do changes the tree itself.

This messed up, imperfect life of mine? It's beautiful. It's a gift.

The Tree of Zoe has the power to bring beauty out of ashes. It has done so for me and it can do so for other teen moms, couples struggling with miscarriage or infertility, women in abusive relationships, people struggling with addiction, parents who aborted their baby, parents who mourn the child they gave up for adoption… anyone and everyone. Life can be dazzling, even with all kinds of heartbreak and scars. The power of zoe is that hope and beauty shine through the imperfections.

I am passionate about choosing and living the zoe life, and my desire to encourage pregnant women to carry their babies to term is a huge part of that. Why? Because a baby changes everything. Two thousand years ago, a baby humbly entered the world, just like every other child before Him: vulnerable, through agony, sweat, blood, and at least a little bit of fear.

It was messy.

It was brutal.

It was beautiful. That baby was named Jesus, and He changed our world and our futures. And nearly four decades ago, a baby named Arica changed mine.

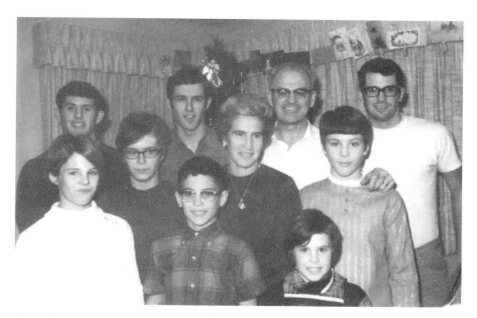

Laura, her parents, and siblings
Christmas, 1967

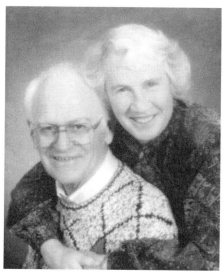

Sally & Richard Hughes
Laura's parents

CHAPTER 2

Baby Bumps

I sat with my hands on the steering wheel at the ten and two positions, just like my dad taught me. I was having a hard time moving my hand toward the key to start the car. I was a bird in a cage, and a moving car was my ticket to freedom. Except I didn't entirely want to leave. For the most part, I really liked my cage—it was wonderful, an aviary. In it were my parents, who had worked so hard and loved me so well, and my marvelous and supportive siblings. But there was danger there too. Bad choices, toxic relationships, a dismal future— they were all part of my life in the cage of Billings, Montana. I had to get out. I had to get *her* out.

I started the car.

As I slowly rolled down our long driveway, spreading my wings for the first time, I took one last look in the rearview mirror. I could see the top of Arica's head as she sat singing softly in the back seat, but beyond her I saw my parents, clinging to each other. My mom later told me my dad was saying, "Are you going to let her do it? Are you really going to let her take our baby?"

He didn't know the only reason I had been strong enough to strike out on my own was because of him and the values he had instilled in his children. We were a good Catholic family, so every morning Dad would load all the kids up in our little red bus like the Partridge family to go to morning mass, then gather us together each evening to pray the rosary and for those in our community.

Every.

Single.

Day.

My parents treated us, and those in the community, with respect and love. I had the privilege of watching their faith and value for life on constant display. When someone in need would show up at our door, I can still hear my dad saying to my mother, "Throw on another potato." I've already told you about my mother's volunteer work, but my dad also did his fair share—writing life-affirming articles for the local *Billings Gazette* and supporting the crisis pregnancy center with my mother. Little did they know their own daughter would need its services.

But I did need its services. When that critical, decisive moment arrived, the belief in the sanctity of life that my parents established in our home helped me make a decision for which I will always be grateful. That decision has grown into a vibrant woman, serving her community as a school psychologist and, along with her husband, raising three of my beautiful grandchildren. And it all started with my parents.

My parents were devoted to us children, and I don't remember them ever making us feel shame even when we messed up royally.

Case-in-point: When I was sixteen, I wrecked my dad's car. That would be bad enough, but it was made worse by the knowledge that I had specifically been told not to drive the Malibu, because it had been sold. In fact, my parents were delivering it to Denver the very next day. But this was an emergency! My friends' car had broken down at the roller-skating rink, and they needed me to pick them up. Like any good friend, I answered the call, despite going against my parents' instruction. Oh, but it gets worse. What did I hit? My church…and school. You read that right. I ran into the corner of the Holy Rosary Church, where I attended high school. What are the chances?

Crawling out the window, I made my way to a pay phone.

"Dad, I just wrecked the Malibu," I squeaked into the receiver.

"Praise the Lord!" he replied.

Really?

"Dad, why can't you get mad like a normal parent?"

"Well, you are calling me, so *you* must be okay. And *it* is just a car."

That was his first reaction, and it was a gift. He and my mother truly treasured their children. It was the same with my pregnancy. Once they found out, they were supportive and loving, and never once tried to make me feel ashamed. Their parenting motto had not changed: Keep the relationship intact.

I first broke the news to my mother, who advised that she be the one to tell Dad when she picked him up at the airport that evening. Though he had never laid a hand on me, I was certain he would kill me, so when my mom left for the airport, I called my boyfriend to come rescue me. I sat in his car in the church parking lot, trying to gather courage to go home. Finally, at three thirty in the morning I decided to face my fate. Hoping my parents were asleep, I crept through the door—but there was my dad, waiting up for me. He looked lovingly at me through his coke-bottle glasses, and I burst into tears. I'll never forget what happened next. He came over to me and embraced me, whispering grace, "I love you! Mom and I are too old to raise another baby. All I ask is that you pray every day what is best for your baby. Either raise her with our support or give her to a loving couple who are waiting to adopt. Now get to sleep. You have school in a couple of hours." Parenting by grace: My parents were masters. I had not given them enough credit, and I believe many young, scared pregnant women do not give their own parents enough credit either. Children can underestimate the powerful, overriding love that parents have for them, even in the face of disappointment.

Many years after Arica was born, I asked my dad how he could always have such a loving response and how he was able to defend me even though I had behaved in ways that should have brought shame to our family. He replied, "You kids are all a gift from God, and you're on loan to me. So if I'm going to be embarrassed by what the neighbors say, then that's just pride."

It wasn't just words; my parents backed up this philosophy with their actions. When my Catholic school found out I was attending with a baby at home, they tried to expel me. My parents wouldn't stand for it and fought hard to keep me in. They weren't concerned about their reputations; they were concerned about my well-being and future, which equated to the well-being and future of my baby.

Once, I heard my dad in the other room talking to a man who

was either from church or work. "Goodness. She's sixteen and has a kid. What are you going to do?" the man said in a tone equal parts disgust and sympathy.

"I'm proud of Laura and her parenting. Having a baby has brought her great responsibility," my father said, indifferent to the man's attempt to judge his daughter. His words sank deep into my heart. To be valued above the opinion of neighbors, church members, and relatives—that was life-giving. His compassion, mercy, and sacrifice of pride gave me hope. It was the embodiment of zoe.

I wish more parents would embrace this concept when faced with the embarrassment of a child's unplanned pregnancy. Sadly, many of the young women I speak with at Alpha Pregnancy Clinics do not have the same experience. They feel pushed away from their parents at a time when they need them the most. In some cultures, the threat of shame falling on the family name leaves the pregnant woman out in the cold, struggling on her own to find solutions. For others, the disappointment they observe in family members leads them to self-isolate or withdraw into friendships that are far from what their parents would wish.

Tiffany was one of those women. I met her a few years ago at an Alpha Pregnancy Clinic, where she sat with me, fist in the air, proclaiming, "No white Republican man is going to tell me what I have to do with my body!" I could tell you her story, but she tells it so well herself:[1]

It all began in November. I started feeling tired, sick, and queasy—symptoms I would soon get acquainted with, for

*they wouldn't leave for another nine months. After dragging
my boyfriend to a local pharmacy so he could buy me a
pregnancy test, the uneasy feelings only intensified after
it came back positive. I was in disbelief. I was so sure the
pregnancy test had gotten it wrong, because how could I have
gotten pregnant? Nobody thinks it could happen to them until
it happens. I was shocked, distraught, confused, surprised, and
numb.*

*I always thought that if I chose to have children, I
would be financially stable, in a healthy, loving relationship,
graduated from school, and established in my career. I
was absolutely none of those things. I was in an unhealthy
relationship with my boyfriend at the time I got pregnant;
I had just begun working; I was two years into college, and
still living with my parents. I felt I was too irresponsible,
inadequate, and completely unprepared to bring a child into
the world—I was just entering adulthood myself. I felt like I
was trapped in a job I didn't remember signing up for.*

*I felt so alone and lost. I didn't know what to do or
what would be best. Things with my boyfriend were rocky,
and when my parents found out, they were angry and
disappointed and made it very clear they didn't want me to
keep the baby.*

The church has great culpability in this cycle of shame and
secrecy that often leads women to abort. Though a pro-life position
is often proclaimed and ardently defended, women who choose to

keep their unplanned pregnancies are often met with disdain, as are their parents, and the problem is compounded. If churches celebrated women who chose life during unplanned pregnancies, instead of focusing on the sexual sin that brought them to this point, women might be more likely to choose life, and parents less likely to push for abortion. I am not excusing sexual sin by any means, but when a woman gets pregnant, the focus shifts. The new life in her is not a sin; rather, it is a gift.

If we are truly pro-life, we will not shame the women who are courageously risking reputation, career goals, and dreams to bring unplanned life into this world.

I see grace in every child. No matter how they got here, they are a blessing to their parents. There are plenty of men and women engaging in sexual sin who go quietly about their lives, destroying any evidence, but it takes a true act of courage to keep a pregnancy when a woman could choose to hide it through abortion and keep up the façade of righteous living.

Many young women who choose abortion do so out of shame. They are afraid of what their parents, friends, and sadly, faith community will say. We owe it to our young women to do better. We must choose zoe and cultivate compassion for those in need: mercy instead of judgment, encouragement in place of yelling, hope where there once was condemnation. If we are truly pro-life, we will not shame the women who are courageously risking reputation, career goals, and dreams to bring unplanned life into this world.

Tiffany continues:

I had just begun to be involved in church again when I found out I was pregnant. I was finally feeling closer to God and being mentored by mature Christians, and it all just got flipped upside-down. None of the church leaders responded positively, save for one. There were no offers for prayer or guidance, much less support. Most of the church leaders turned away from me and stopped communicating entirely.

In the absence of church support, I turned to my friends. Their response wasn't much better. One even told me I should get an abortion because I wasn't responsible enough. I tried my best to stay strong and keep my ears open for the only opinion I knew mattered—God's. It was a struggle, though, to work through this inner turmoil all on my own.

I had a flawed perception of myself, which was reflected in the fact that I stayed longer in a toxic relationship. How I viewed God also shaped my feelings at the time, as well as the way I was raised by my parents. My community and culture centered around a performance-based mentality, and I imposed that narrative and understanding into my relationship with God as well. I believed I had to be good to be worthy. I felt like I wouldn't be loved or appreciated by my family, friends, and even God if I wasn't constantly making good decisions.

I contemplated abortion. It just seemed like the easiest route. No one would need to know. My image could stay intact.

Image was an overriding theme in my own life. Though my family did not shame me, shame crept in—largely from my molestation, but also from church, society, and school—and held me captive. When I discovered I was pregnant, the guilt and shame of my situation prevented me from telling anyone and getting the help I needed for almost six months. Thankfully, my family did not meet my expectations, but rather showed me grace and mercy, which in turn gave me courage and a chance to truly consider my options.

Once my mom found out about my pregnancy, she took me to the family doctor I had seen since infancy. You know, the one I was too embarrassed to even tell I had started my menstrual cycle. Lovely. Knowing I was the youngest of eight from a good Irish Catholic family, naturally he had an adoptive family all lined up. I went to some adoption agencies and looked through the binders of prospective families to appease my parents. It was the first time I truly considered how brave and sacrificial a woman had to be to place her child for adoption. I developed a deep respect for those women, but I knew I wanted to keep my baby.

I'm grateful that my parents didn't push me one way or the other. They presented the options of adoption or of keeping my baby, and they let me know they would support me in my decision. Because they had instilled a strong belief in the sanctity of life, I never even considered abortion.

Women today are bombarded with the message that abortion is often the best, if not only, option when dealing with an unplanned pregnancy. They are told that the thing growing inside them is the source of their anxiety, that they may face embarrassment, shunning, and the end of their dreams for the future. They are told to destroy it and their problems will go away. They are told they will suffer no physical or mental side effects. And most loudly, they are told it is their body and that they should only think of themselves.

If the first place a woman facing an unplanned pregnancy turns when searching for answers is online, the nation's leading abortion provider's website will greet her with an overtly biased message. The three options for pregnancy—abortion, adoption, and parenting— are listed in obvious preferential order, with abortion being the best, simplest choice, adoption being doable with pain involved, and parenting being all but a death sentence.

If the counseling women receive in these clinics is as overtly biased as the website, it is no wonder the numbers of abortions are so high and adoption referrals so low.

In the 2014-2015 fiscal year, only 2,062 referrals for adoption were given, contrasted with 323,999 abortion procedures performed (and that doesn't include prescriptions for at-home medical abortions).[2] It is clear where the abortion industry's leading provider places its focus, regardless of the cloak of "women's healthcare."

If the first place a woman facing an unplanned pregnancy turns when searching for answers is online, the nation's leading abortion provider's website will greet her with an overtly biased message. The three options for pregnancy—abortion, adoption, and parenting—are listed in obvious preferential order, with abortion being the best, simplest choice, adoption being doable with pain involved, and parenting being all but a death sentence.

It makes me so sad to think of women who buy into the lie that abortion is their only option and who walk a very lonely path at abortion clinics, where little to no follow up care is provided. At the crisis pregnancy center where I volunteer, we regularly see women suffering from the effects of abortion—both physical and emotional. And while it would not serve the abortion movement well to acknowledge it, *we* are the ones who help these women find a path to healing.

Pregnancy resource centers are an excellent place to start when facing an unplanned pregnancy. Below are support services offered in communities across the United States:

- Information and education, including free pregnancy tests and ultrasounds to help women make an informed decision about their pregnancies.[3]
- Medical referrals and prenatal care.

- STI testing and treatment.
- Emotional support for those who have chosen an abortion or experienced a miscarriage or stillbirth.
- Counseling to explore best options for a mother and her baby based on her circumstances.
- Resource assistance, such as housing, education, or medical services.
- Cohesive parental support for both mothers and fathers, through parenting classes, breastfeeding instruction, early childhood development, and instruction on safe practices to lower the risk of Sudden Infant Death Syndrome (SIDS).
- Tangible support, such as diapers, cribs, and other necessities.
- Help with adoption processes as needed. [ii]

By God's grace, the counsel at Liberty Church, and the dedicated ministry of Alpha Pregnancy Clinics of Northern California, Tiffany's story doesn't end the way it does for so many women facing their unplanned pregnancy alone:

> *My boyfriend and I were connected to Liberty Church,*
> *where we received counseling. One of the main pastors*
> *counseled women post-abortion, and she gave me information*
> *on early fetal development, as well as talked to us about our*
> *options. She mentioned that Alpha Pregnancy Clinic offered*

---

ii   For more information about available options for women facing unplanned pregnancies, see Appendix A at the back of this book.

free and confidential services for women who were in my situation.

After a few more nights wrestling with feeling scared and alone, I decided to make an appointment. What did I have to lose?

I came into Alpha still unsure of how they would be able to help or where to start. Kathy met me at the front desk and was so kind and welcoming, and I spoke with Laura, who genuinely cared about my situation. Not only did she listen to what I had to say, she shared about similar feelings she had being pregnant at a young age and then told me where her life was now. Listening to Laura talk was inspiring and encouraging; it reminded me that everything was going to turn out all right in the end. I continued to speak with Laura, and when it got more difficult to drive all the way up to the pregnancy center, she made time to speak with me weekly on the phone. She would chat with me and be a friend and listening ear when I needed it most.

She gave me hope that I wasn't alone, that I was going to be okay.

When I finally had my first official prenatal check-up, I was already beginning to think that an abortion would have a traumatic effect on me. But when I actually saw my baby on the ultrasound…I was speechless. She was so tiny; the doctor could barely point her out. Even when the doctor had left the room, I had a million thoughts bombarding my mind, but still, words had failed me. I then burst into tears, unable to control the overflow of emotion. I realized I couldn't let my little one down. It wasn't going to be easy, but I knew it would be worth it.

On July 4, at 11:24 a.m., I was blessed with a beautiful baby girl named Alaska Rose.

According to Tiffany, Alpha Pregnancy Clinics of Northern California saved her future by saving her daughter's. Ironically, according to one prominent abortion provider website, women should be leery of crisis and pregnancy resource centers because, "These fake clinics seem like medical centers that offer abortions or other pregnancy options, but they're actually run by people who want to scare or shame people out of getting an abortion."[4] Let me set the record straight: Pregnancy resource centers are known for their compassion and lack of shaming (just talk to someone who has been to one). They do *not* put on the guise of offering abortions, but *do* offer other pregnancy options—everything but abortion, in fact. The implication of this quote is so skewed it is almost funny: Apparently, *all* the "other pregnancy options" that these centers *do* offer don't count. To them, abortion is the only true option.

I have also heard the "fake clinic" claim with my own ears. Through a series of events, I was invited to volunteer at a large convention of abortion advocates. At first I shuddered at the thought, but eventually my curiosity, sense of justice, and prayerful consideration prevailed, and I found myself signing in guests for a VIP reception and later attending a breakout session on "fake clinics."

I sat quietly taking notes on all the easily disproved arguments they had against pregnancy centers, fighting the urge to shed light on the fallibility of their statements. An abortion doctor made the claim that pregnancy centers switch out ultrasounds to scare women into parenting. He suggested they show a woman who is seven weeks pregnant the ultrasound of a woman who is twenty weeks pregnant. I almost snorted.

How gullible does he think women are? I thought.

The speaker continued by denigrating Abby Johnson, a former abortion clinic staffer who left the industry and exposed its morally corrupt inner-workings. Today, she helps others do the same with her book, *Unplanned*, and ministry, And Then There Were None.[5]

After scoffing at Abby and those like her, the speaker went on to lament how "fake clinics" pop up in the same communities where "real clinics" already exist and that the fake clinics are targeting low-income and minority neighborhoods.

Wait. Who did she say was in those neighborhoods first?

In light of their claim of "fake clinics," it seems odd that an organization so dedicated to women's health only provided a mere 17,419 prenatal services, a paltry fraction of one percent of its over nine million services for the year. Apparently, women who would normally use their clinics for services had to go to the "fake" pregnancy centers to get the prenatal help they needed, because the women's health clinics had little use for them if they weren't going to pay for an abortion.

I am proud to serve at a so-called "fake clinic," because they offer so much to the community. But there are also other options for women with unplanned pregnancies. Another excellent option for women in this position is the Public Health Department. Counties vary in services provided, but some have robust programs. Beth Jones is a nurse with Nurse-Family Partnership, a non-profit organization designed to help low-income, first-time mothers (those who have never had a live birth). In her work, she partners one-on-one with women during weekly or bi-weekly meetings to improve pregnancy outcomes, monitor their health, and provide parenting resources. Once a baby is born, she continues her visits for two years, providing physical assessments and resources to improve child development and parenting self-sufficiency. The program also connects parents to other resources in their community, whether it be counseling or the need for financial assistance through programs such as Women, Infants, and Children (WIC) or Cash Aid.

According to Beth, studies have shown that a window of time exists for first-time mothers to break out of old patterns or parenting styles they experienced as children and make real and positive change for their own children. The Nurse-Family Partnership program aims to capitalize on this window to help mothers successfully and healthily raise the next generation. For low-income women who are scared at the prospect of being a parent, this in-depth, personal help may be just what they need.[6]

Forty years ago, there weren't as many options for pregnant teens like me. Thankfully, I had the support of my family. My parents accepted my decision to keep Arica, but the rest of society did not. Due to some insurance glitch, my birthing expenses wouldn't be covered if I lived with my parents, so I spent the summer leading up to Arica's arrival living with my sister over two hours away in

Bozeman. Because of the distance and a quick delivery, my parents didn't arrive until after Arica was born. During the interim, the hospital staff tried to keep her from me, hoping that a failure to bond would make me more inclined to put her up for adoption. When my parents did finally arrive, the pediatrician looked at my mother and said, "How could you let her go through with this pregnancy? Why didn't you have her abort?" Not exactly the affirming words a new mother is looking for.

Luckily, the atmosphere was different at home. I can still picture walking into a room and seeing my dad bouncing Arica on his knee, his pop-bottle glasses hardly able to hide the twinkle in his eyes. Every morning she would be there, snuggled on his lap as he read his Bible. And the first thing he'd do when he got home from work was swoop her up so he and my mom could sing her silly kids songs. Their love and acceptance for her spoke volumes of their love and acceptance for me.

One of the greatest things my parents did for us kids was stand beside us during our struggles, but not fix them for us. Plenty of grandparents raise their grandchildren, but my parents would not be counted among them. They supported me and loved me but made it clear from the beginning that parenting had been my choice and that they were too old to start over again. They didn't leave me to flounder on my own, though. Parenting eight children had taught them a thing or two. "Inconsistency is the enemy of good parenting," my dad used to say. "You can't put her in time out one time and then pop her in the butt or yell at her the next. Choose wisely, and then be consistent."

They also taught me the importance of putting her down at a

regular time, because "every adult needs a little time to herself."

Adult. I loved that he acknowledged I had moved to a different place in my life, even if I wasn't yet fully grown. That said, they understood I was still a teen and wanted to be with my friends, who were also teens. Once I put Arica down for the night, I was allowed to go out, as long as I was home by 9:30 p.m. in order to get a good night's rest for school.

The subject my parents had the strongest opinion about was that of my school attendance. Continuing school and graduating was non-negotiable, and they did what they could to create a safe environment where I could do so. They provided me with a car so I could take Arica to my sister's in the morning on my way to school, and they advocated for me as issues arose. They helped with Arica so I could be in the school play, then proudly attended and cheered me on. The parenting habits and boundaries they set for me were all influenced by that end: I must graduate. In our town, dropping out of high school was almost a life sentence for poverty, and that wasn't an option for a prized daughter and granddaughter. They sought to build me up as a young lady, helping me with my first job interview and encouraging me to participate in activities that gave me confidence. They pushed me to still achieve my dreams. I knew that whatever happened, they would be fair and treat me with dignity.

When Arica was one, I had a dream that showed me the miserable future that awaited Arica and me if I stayed in Billings. I was stuck in an unhealthy, unfaithful relationship, and I seemed incapable of being resolute in ending it. It became clear to me that the only solution was to leave and get far beyond the reach of my boyfriend and my emotional attachment to him. We had a close family friend living in California, so I decided Arica and I would start over there. Even though it broke their hearts to let us go, my parents' support never wavered.

As hard as it was, I'm convinced leaving that toxic relationship saved us. I know there are many women in similar relationships who can't see a way out. But my heart's cry is that we show them there truly is. They are *not* alone. I long for the day when we have embraced the zoe life in our families and churches in such a way that a woman facing an unplanned pregnancy will want to turn there first, not be terrified at the prospect. I want us to love our children so well and completely that they know we will walk through these scary paths with them. I want multigenerational communities to come alongside these women and honor their decision to keep life and offer to mentor and help. I want godly families and churches to be the place where women are set free from their shame and the pain of the past that has driven them into desperate situations.

I want us to reach out with a helping hand to women (and men!) who have chosen life and might be struggling. The battle was not simply won when birth was chosen over abortion.

Choosing zoe means partnering with these parents to help them be successful. That could take on many forms. For example: babysitting so they can attend school or parenting classes or get a much-needed break; providing a meal so they can have time with their child while juggling work, school, or single parenting; helping to provide financially for necessities; being a mentor and parenting coach. Bottom line: If we are truly pro-life, we will care for these babies before *and* after they are born.

We must have more than empathy; we must have compassion. Empathy is feeling with a person, but compassion takes it one step further—along with feeling, it believes there is a better way, and it isn't content to simply feel along with a person in their desperate state.[7] It cries for action, for change! We can be that change. We are surrounded by women who need that change. When the world sees the compassion that healthy, whole families and churches have for women in crisis pregnancies, it can't help but have a ripple effect.

Bottom line: If we are truly pro-life, we will care for these babies before *and* after they are born.

Failure in the past does not condemn our futures. We serve a God of grace and forgiveness. He is there for the woman in crisis pregnancy. He is there for the woman who has had an abortion. And He is there for the families and churches who have failed these women. God is a God of second chances, and Tiffany is living proof:

> *My friend was right: I wasn't responsible enough to raise a baby. But if anybody ever says they are, they're lying.*
> *What do you have to do and in what place in your life do you have to be in order to feel completely ready to take on a whole new life for the rest of yours? Married? Financially*

stable? Those things may make it easier, but if you ask me, nothing in life prepares you for the crazy journey of parenthood. It takes courage, maturity, and a great deal of selflessness to raise a child. We all fail in one area or another. But parenting isn't about perfection, and I try my best.

Alpha gave me hope and perseverance when I thought I was at the end of my rope. Coming to Alpha allowed me to realize there was no perfect pregnancy story and that women are in various places and struggle with different things. They taught me that there can be compassion and support without judgment when you really need it, and I am so appreciative of them for that.

This experience was a turning point in my spiritual life as well. I realized God does not demand perfection. He never withheld His unconditional love from me. He loves me the same on my worst days as He does on my best. Jesus didn't come for the perfect; He came for the sick. Without pain and heartbreak, we would never feel the need to reach out to Jesus's outstretched arms or surrender to His powerful love.

Though the rejection from my church could have had terrible consequences, I've been able to forgive and understand that everybody grows up with a different narrative of who God is. Although they may be deeply involved in the church, their understanding of God may be rooted in religion rather than the loving, forgiving, compassionate grace of Jesus Christ. I am now blessed with a church that constantly showers Alaska and me with love and help—from babysitting so I can finish my degree, to giving us a Christmas tree complete with presents.

Starting out as a single parent with no savings has been hard. There have been times when I didn't know where we'd get our next meal. I work long hours, attend school, and try to be both mom and dad to this sweet little person. But…the bond it has created is also our greatest gift. We have learned to treasure the small things and each other. I am so blessed to be her mother.

To the woman facing an unplanned pregnancy, I won't lie to you. The road ahead will be hard at times. There will be struggles left and right, and some days you will cry into your pillow and hope it all ends. But in the morning, the sun will shine again. Faith isn't a brightly shining sun whose rays are felt at all times of the day. Sometimes the fog and clouds get in the way, but it doesn't mean the sun has ever left us. Cling to the love of Jesus Christ. He is the only Redeemer. I may have to surrender several times a day, but these are always the best decisions I make. To parents of someone facing an unplanned pregnancy—love her and support her. She may not want to hear guidance and advice, but she will need the love and encouragement from her loved ones more than anything during this time. My own parents will tell you that they did not want me to carry out this pregnancy, but now that they have met Alaska, they can't imagine their lives without one of their greatest blessings. To the faith community—reach out to women in crisis pregnancy with support and kind words. Do all things in love. Be compassionate, the way Jesus was to all.

Chapter 2

There is no amount of pain that Jesus cannot handle.
Let Him take it, let Him free your heavy burdens. We are all
beautifully and wonderfully made.

Arica's birth began a new chapter in my life and provided me with a second (and third, and fourth…) chance. But there were echoes from the previous chapter of my life that had to be dealt with first. Clearly, my pregnancy was the culmination of issues that began much earlier.

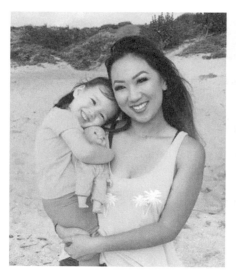

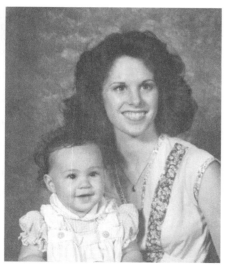

Tiffany & daughter Alaska Rose

Laura & Arica at age 1

CHAPTER 3

Of Sex and Hearses

The car stank. Actually, that is too nice of a word—it *reeked*. When I had asked a family friend for a ride from where I was living with my sister in Bozeman to my home back in Billings, Montana, I hadn't given much thought to his line of work.

I should have.

Our friend owned a chain of funeral homes, and on this particular day, he was using his hearse to transport the body of a man who had died three days earlier to Billings for cremation. Holding my breath while the driver chain-smoked, I rolled the window down and put my hand out to let the air turn my arm into an airplane moving in the turbulence. My long hair fluttered around me, and wisps kept tickling my nose and creeping into my eyes as I squinted into the scorching summer sun. In front of me, the Absaroka Mountains rose to meet the sky, undaunted by its vast expanse and impervious to the nauseating smell from the corpse behind me. There was only one thing that had made me load my eight-months pregnant belly into that hearse for the two-and-a-half-hour drive: my boyfriend. Being away from him was torture. Was he thinking about me as much as I was of him? I was desperate to find out.

At the time, the love I felt for my boyfriend was the one thing I wished my parents understood about me, but we didn't discuss such things in my house. Here I was, fifteen years old and eight months pregnant, yet sex and my relationship with my boyfriend was a topic that didn't come up. Part of the communication barricade was generational, and part of it was the religious culture in which we lived. I often wonder how different my life would have been if my parents and I had a relationship in which we had been open to discussing those kinds of things. Perhaps my parents wanted to dialogue about it with me, but by the time I was fifteen, they didn't feel they could. We had not built the type of relationship that made any of us comfortable chatting about taboo topics. I remember one of the few times my mother directly mentioned my pregnancy.

We were driving in the car when she said, "Your father comes home from his business trip tonight. I'm going to tell him you are pregnant when I pick him up at the airport."

Silence.

She glanced over at me for a second, then turned her eyes back to the road. I kept staring out the window instead of looking at her, my breath making a little opaque circle on the glass. Thoughts whirled in my head. What could I say? That I was ashamed of myself, but despite that shame I was excited to be pregnant? That I'd seen other people in my family get pregnant out of wedlock and go on to have happy marriages, so of course I would too? That I wish I hadn't slept with my boyfriend, but didn't necessarily plan on stopping? No words would change the situation, so I sat, mute. I suppose we had become accustomed to these uncomfortable silences.

She sighed. With no ping-pong of conversation, my mother let it drop. She may have been testing the waters for intimacy, but the "No Swimming" sign had been posted prominently for so many years that I didn't dare jump in with her.

With the emergence of the phrase "emotional intelligence" in 1990, its subsequent popularity, and the self-awareness of current Millennials, families today are more open about such topics—at least to a point—and this is a step in the right direction. Still, cultural and environmental variances ensure that every family will have a different comfort level discussing sexual issues. Parents need not move beyond age-appropriate material to establish a sense of trust with their children.

I am not suggesting they speak in indecorous ways or promote flippant attitudes toward sex. I would encourage families, however, to discern their children's emotional readiness and to push past discomfort for their betterment. As parents, we are the strongest advocates for our kids. If they can't come to us to ask the important and embarrassing questions, they will go to someone else—someone who does not treasure them the way we do and perhaps won't share our same core values and beliefs.

So, how and when to begin? First, I think it is critical that parents make the effort to work through their own junk if they want their children to feel safe working through theirs. Many problems children face, and the manifestations they have, are in direct measure to their parents' issues. If children are exhibiting problems, it may be most beneficial for parents to first receive counseling. A rebellious teen may simply feel disconnected from her parents, but once she *feels* loved, the rebellion will diminish.

Once parents have confronted their own issues, then they are ready to help their children. If parents wait until they have a teenager before creating a culture of openness, safety, and trust, it may be too late. From the moment a child learns to speak, parents are provided with ample opportunity to establish that intimacy. It starts with the little things. These things may seem insignificant on their own, but built upon each other, they create a safe place for a child to discuss increasingly complex issues. The following ideas are not exhaustive, but they are a starting place.

- Engage in your children's everyday activities. For instance, ask specific questions that get real answers about their time at school and with friends, paying special attention when they seem like they've had a difficult day, changed emotionally, or are acting out. What happened? How did it make them feel? Is there something they could have done differently? Do they need to talk to someone other than you about what happened—a teacher, authority figure, counselor, or peer?

- In this process, always measure their heart. Ask them, "How's your heart doing today?" If they don't already, they'll begin to trust you with their heart and learn to express themselves. "My heart feels sad, lonely, scared...." When you are able, dig deeper:

"Why do you think that is? How could we make your heart feel better or safer?"

- Acknowledge the validity of children's concerns, even when they seem silly.
- Do not share private stories or pictures about them they would find embarrassing with other parents or on social media.
- Allow them to ask questions without making them feel foolish, even when their questions make you feel uncomfortable.
- Keep your word, regardless if it's inconvenient.
- Don't be hypocritical—children need to see core values modeled for them. For instance, if you teach them that gossiping is wrong, then they should never hear you gossip. Make sure your words match your actions, and pay close attention to your interactions with others. If you are married, your children will develop their own interactions based on those between you and your spouse.
- Ask what they think about certain topics, don't belittle or shame them for that opinion, and use the opportunity to celebrate how God made them different than you.
- Admit when you are wrong, and if need be, apologize.
- Confess some of your failings so they can see that failure is part of learning and won't affect their status in the family.
- Be an example of vulnerability. When the time comes, the level of vulnerability and openness you have had in your daily life will equal the level of vulnerability and openness your child feels discussing sex and other difficult topics.

Another avenue parents can use to create openness around this subject is to attend previews offered by the school system of the Sex Education curriculum. Our Alpha Prevention[8] team offers such previews at various schools, and I am always amazed at how few parents show up. (When my own school held such an event, my mother was the only one who went.) It is unfortunate, both because we offer talking points that parents can use with their kids—the fact that the number of Sexually Transmitted Diseases (STDs) has increased from four to twenty in one generation, the amazing stages of fetal development that point to life at conception, good ways to prevent teen pregnancy—and because this would help parents keep tabs on what their child is learning.

But how to bring up the uncomfortable topic of sex, especially when you are from a reserved background or a family who never discussed such things? Being factual about the body and how it works is a natural starting point and begins when children are young. This allows children to feel comfortable discussing their bodies and related topics from an early age. While many programs advocate teaching children the actual names for their anatomy to help identify and protect from sexual exploitation, I would suggest that it also demystifies the conversations surrounding human sexuality. This, in turn, gives parents a practical and scientific base for understanding the body, upon which they can build spiritual and moral lessons regarding self-worth and personal conduct.

If children can learn to esteem the human body, then they will hopefully be more likely to discuss body-related issues openly. Because of our own embarrassment on the subject, we sometimes inadvertently teach children that their bodies, especially their sexual organs, are dirty or bad, and thus create shame around any topic related to them. This is unfortunate. Puberty is a critical and difficult time of development, and children need their parents to help them navigate these unchartered waters. Children and teens are curious, and sadly, they are bombarded by an overly sexualized culture. If parents are unwilling to discuss these matters, for example, not answering what a sexual term means, kids will find someone who is, or they will turn to the internet and likely find illicit material that can profoundly affect their developing psyches. If that happens, not only has the parent lost a chance to bond with a child and increase trust, they have missed an opportunity to create context and give moral guidance. Conversely, if parents have built a culture of trust and honesty with children during their younger years, a culture where vulnerability and questioning is encouraged, then chances are they will be the ones their children go to when issues arise or a life-altering decision needs to be made.

When teens are pregnant, the first place they go is usually their do-or-die moment. If they choose the prevailing women's health clinic that performs abortions, or a friend who has had an abortion, they will most likely have an abortion. If instead they have a safe place where they know there will be unconditional support, they are given the gift of time to pause, ponder, and make a rational decision.

I wish I could say that I learned from my experience and did a better job with my own children. However, childhood and convention die hard. My children wanted to discuss sex and relationships with me, but it was embarrassing. It made me feel uncomfortable, so I shut them down, and they suffered as a result. I have no doubt that the subconscious pain and shame from the abuse I suffered, coupled with having sex with my boyfriend so young, were contributing factors to my silence. As with much of this book, I do not come from a place of perfection and success. I am building things out of my mess. I handled such topics the way my parents did, as did their parents before them. It is hard to break generational influence and patterns. We must cultivate our emotional intelligence and discover why we do the things we do and then be humble enough to implement a better way, if there is one.

When teens are pregnant, the first place they go is usually their do-or-die moment. If they choose the prevailing women's health clinic that performs abortions, or a friend who has had an abortion, they will most likely have an abortion. If instead they have a safe place where they know there will be unconditional support, they are given the gift of time to pause, ponder, and make a rational decision.

I have learned lessons, sometimes slowly, and have become a better person from them. The same is true for all parents. Some feel that mistakes in their past have taken away their capacity to teach and guide on certain issues. Nothing could be further from the truth. What better voice than one who has been through the trenches and can articulate the consequences? This is where that established vulnerability comes into play again. When we are honest about the things we've done and what it feels like to have a broken heart or wounded soul, our kids will find us to be even more approachable. No longer are we people who can be easily dismissed with unattainable expectations. We are human, just like them. Parents don't have to air every bit of dirty laundry, but having a few pieces on the line will add credence to our perspective.

Parents who are joyful and embrace their faith and the zoe life, regardless of past mistakes, offer something refreshing to their families. God doesn't need us to hide our mistakes. If He did, the Bible would be very short indeed and only filled with happy stories. Instead, it is fraught with blood, guts, rape, and murder. Repeatedly, the children of Israel are told to learn from their forefathers' mistakes. When our children see us acknowledge our mistakes, they will be less apt to hide theirs. Breaking a generational cycle of problems and addictions is my goal. I was not prepared with my children, but I have gained knowledge on the Alpha Prevention team and am now equipped to teach my grandchildren. All is not lost; redemption is possible. We are never too old to learn and instill blessing.

As a teen, I had no idea about hormones. I was so embarrassed about puberty-related issues that I lied to my mom and family doctor for years because I didn't want to discuss what was happening with my body. When I first kissed a boy, the physiological response took me by complete surprise. I felt things in places I had never felt them before. I became light-headed and confused—it was wonderful! I wanted more. But I was unprepared, and in my innocence I assumed that rush of emotion had to be love. Perhaps I would have made the same choices, but I can't help but think I would have been wiser if I had been armed with knowledge and a solid biblical framework beyond simply, "The Bible says sex before marriage is a sin. Don't have sex."

I was too young and ill-equipped to understand all facets of love on my own. I didn't understand that God made us this way for marriage and sex by creating our limbic system, which gets activated when we fall in love. Our brain is rewarded with dopamine. God designed us this way so the earth will be filled with His image. My adult lens sees clearly how I confused sex with love. Now I see I am wired for love.

Teens get stuck in physically unhealthy relationships because sex is powerful. The physiological reaction and release of oxytocin that happens during intercourse was created to bond a man and woman for life. When used as a drug, out of context, it wreaks havoc.

As marriage and family therapists and pastors, Barry and Lori Byrne describe love as having three legs: spiritual oneness, emotional oneness, and sexual oneness. All three are needed for healthy romantic love. The church is good about dealing with the spiritual and emotional aspects, while not giving enough emphasis to the sexual realm. We shy away from topics regarding sex and downplay its importance, perhaps to reduce interest on the part of those who are not married. Teens are often not taught that God cares a great deal about their desire for sex and to be loved. On the other end of the spectrum, our culture places almost all the emphasis on sex and shuns the other two legs. Media creates an unrealistic view of sex and fuels desires that have no righteous outlet outside of marriage. We need to teach young people the full depth of what a relationship can be: something far greater than sex.

Teens get stuck in physically unhealthy relationships because sex is powerful. The physiological reaction and release of oxytocin that happens during intercourse was created to bond a man and woman for life. When used as a drug, out of context, it wreaks havoc.

The Byrnes explain it this way:

When you are in a state of heightened sexual arousal, feelings are not your friend. You need something outside of yourself to pull you out of it. You need an understanding of your self-worth, a spiritual pull greater than your feelings, or someone who is rooting for you and your sexual purity. Feelings distort reality and hide truth.

Sex is far more than a chemical response, for it carries with it a supernatural component. It is the glue that binds a couple together and helps them go through life as one. When this powerful, sacred act is performed outside of the covenant of marriage—from pure sexual desire rather than the devotion to live a life with someone—it is corrupted and defiled. The Bible says in 2 Corinthians 6:14 that we should not be unequally yoked. The image here is of two beasts of burden being joined by a wooden yoke, essentially stuck together, in order to commence agricultural work as a team. Together they can pull heavier equipment and make greater progress than they could on their own. The analogy is perfect for marriage. I remember my dad telling me this as a teen, though I didn't grasp it at the time. God doesn't want us to stick ourselves to someone with whom we don't plan to journey through life. Teens who have sex outside of marriage often say they feel like they are being ripped apart when they aren't with the person or when the relationship is over. Well, that is because they metaphorically *are* being torn. They stuck themselves to someone with the glue of sex without building the necessary spiritual and emotional foundation to sustain a life-long relationship, and tearing something apart that has been glued together is difficult, damaging, and painful.[9] The oxytocin released during intercourse is the same chemical released when a mother breastfeeds her baby. In both cases, it is a glue meant for lasting relationships. Since the word *oxytocin* begins with *ox*, I always think of "being stuck together for life" when I hear it.

The duct tape activity we use in our Alpha abstinence program has connected with teens both in the United States and abroad and illustrates well the "stickiness" of sex. During the presentation, teen volunteers come forward, and we place a piece of duct tape on them. Volunteers are then asked to remove their tape and place it on someone else. As the tape gets passed around, lint from clothing, tack from different tape pieces, and other residue begins to adhere to the tape, and it eventually no longer sticks well. The students are grossed out thinking about picking up potential STDs when "sticking" to multiple sexual partners, but they also clearly see how such behavior can affect their ability to bond once they have lost their "stickiness."

An argument I often hear when advocating for sexual abstinence outside of marriage is that God gave us a sex drive. Either we should be able to use it as it was given, or God is on some sort of mean-spirited power trip to withhold pleasure. Again, the Byrnes:

> *Sexual temptation does not cease to exist once one is married. Men and women must continue to fight against this seduction in order to keep the marriage pure. An excellent training ground for practicing this restraint is by maintaining pure sexual boundaries prior to marriage. Thus, self-control in the sexual arena prior to marriage prepares you for self-control within the marriage. God gives us hormones before He gives us a mate. He does that on purpose so that we can learn to live with the tension of desire and self-control. None of it is to be mean.*

Now, back to the hearse. I endured that long, pungent ride because I had given my heart and body to a boy. I thought I was being rational. When I finally arrived, sweat dripped off my red face onto the welcome mat at the doorway. Dad waved at the driver, and then looked at me pitifully and said, "If I had known you wanted to come home that badly, I would have come and gotten you myself." I sat in my favorite green velvet chair, feeling the fan blow on me and envisioning my reunion with my boyfriend. When my mom finally pulled up in my getaway car—an old Renault our family had affectionately dubbed *Renetta*—I was more than ready to get to his house.

Love lasted in my family, so I believed ours would too, especially since I was the mother of his child. When I arrived at his house, I was rewarded for my efforts by discovering that he was out with another girl. I was friends with his sister, so I stayed there until he got home. I tried to pretend that he was happy to see me and that the other girl wasn't still outside yelling obscenities at me through the screen door. I remember sitting there at his kitchen table, twirling spaghetti on my fork, while he ignored me and I ignored her. I was heartbroken. This wasn't how it was supposed to be. I rationalized reasons he wouldn't want to have me, but nothing could explain why he wouldn't want his own baby. It was almost too much to bear. Yet, somehow, I did bear it, and I kept going back for more.

Looking back, it's hard to believe I continued for so long in a relationship in which I was so poorly treated. I was not ready for sex. I believe the main reason I allowed myself to be devalued and had such a low self-esteem stemmed from my molestation, but I think it was also due, in part, to my desire for physical affection from a male. My dad had always been affectionate with us when we were little, but as we approached puberty, he stopped. Years later he told my sister it was because he had been taught it was inappropriate after a certain age. In retrospect, he realized his mistake, and it made him sad. A growing body of research shows the importance of parent-teen physical affection.[10] Children who lack physical affection at home act out more often in school, are at an increased risk of teenage pregnancy, have a higher school drop-out rate, and exhibit difficulty establishing intimacy in future relationships.[11]

This is disheartening news for some parents since children often begin to withdraw from physical contact around this age. The perceived need to seem mature by shunning parental touch, coupled with the remaining desire for such affection, can help to explain why teens struggle so greatly with failed early relationships. Having rejected physical affection from parents, they fill the need with a romantic partner. When they no longer have it from either, they feel a double loss. This seems to hit teen boys especially hard due to the fact that, unlike their female counterparts, they are less likely to have formed affectionate platonic relationships.

This advice is all well and good, but what happens when you have followed parenting guidance and had the best intentions to protect your children, and the plan you had for your child's life still doesn't go the way you thought it would? Your child chose to become sexually active, and you can't understand why. Perhaps you tried to establish a relationship of honesty and trust too late instead of early. It could be that outside influences led them away from their childhood instruction. Maybe they endured pain and trauma, possibly about which you knew nothing.

There are a myriad of reasons why lives take detours, and none of them automatically indict you as being a bad parent. Nor, for that matter, do they condemn your child. Within the process below, do everything in your power to find out what happened. If your child endured trauma, you need to know about it. I wish my parents had known about my molestation. Early intervention could have made a huge difference in my life. What I would have given not to have waited four decades to find healing. I am so grateful that our society is more proactive about discussing improper touch with children and that parents are more aware of what signs to look for. But we must remain vigilant. Too often we seek to find solutions to the symptoms, such as nightmares or bedwetting, but not the cause. Our kids are counting on us to be their advocates, because they may not even know how to process what has happened to them.

The Byrnes note that sex is often an easy way to satisfy pain and a lack of value. Those who have a healthy understanding of their self-worth are typically quick to recognize people in their lives who manipulate, take advantage, and perpetuate pain. Of course, the opposite is also true. People who allow themselves to be repeatedly mistreated in relationships likely hold very little regard for their self-worth. Parents need to pray for a spiritual breakthrough for their teens, as well as for wisdom on how to better love and guide them through their brokenness. Teens do not typically have enough emotional intelligence to do this on their own. They need a parent, a trusted godly friend or adult, or perhaps even a Christian counselor to journey with them.

The Byrnes have some helpful advice on how to proceed:

> *First, you need to understand that teens who think they are in love and have connected sexually are not usually rational. Second, you are competing with something they feel strongly, and if you lecture or shame, you are making it*

easy for them to justify denying what God says. As always, prayer should be your first resource. Once you have bathed the situation in prayer, spend more time asking questions than you do talking. Get them thinking about their situation by asking things such as:

- *Have you thought about what this relationship will lead to?*
- *Have you thought about the risks of sex outside of marriage?*
- *How well do you know this person?*
- *Have you thought about a future with them? Is this person your life partner?*
- *How will you feel if this relationship doesn't last?*
- *How have things been changed by having sex?*
- *How do you feel about yourself?*
- *Will he or she be a good parent to your future children?*

If you find there is no way to reason with your teen, immerse yourself again in prayer. Declare who they are and the purity of what they are called to be. Pray for their future as a husband or wife, mother or father. God doesn't want His plan for their life to be aborted by their lust, feelings, and pain. Pray that God shows you how to discover any pain they may have experienced.

In our work, we often find that what on the outside appears to be lust can actually be depression or a coping mechanism for pain. Inviting in the Spirit of Truth (another

name for the Holy Spirit), and exploring the reason behind
the perceived lust or sexual promiscuity can bring much
healing. Help your child break the denial of past pain and
work through the grief. You may need to help your children
overcome feelings of shame or guilt for putting themselves in a
bad situation. Getting children to open up and not stay hidden
in their pain is the first step, and they must feel safe to do so.
Depending on your teen's level of pain or trauma, you may feel
overwhelmed or underequipped. Together, explore the idea of
enlisting the help of a Christian counselor.

I would be remiss if I did not say this last word on premarital sex. While sex outside the marriage covenant is serious and carries with it consequences, the church has done harm with the notion that such an act spells doom for future relationships. A teen does not have to relinquish hope of a successful marriage just because they messed up. Yes, it has been complicated and there will be issues to work through and strong emotional ties to break, but God can still forgive and bring fullness. If those who engage in premarital sex are told their future is hopeless or that they are somehow now made unworthy of a godly spouse, their self-worth declines, continuing the vicious circle. Whatever pain, shame, isolation, or depression drove them to make those choices will only be increased. The problems will only grow, and the relationship with our children will continue to deteriorate. We must do better by our children. We must rise above the personal pain and sorrow we feel at their choice and continue our God-given calling to be their stewards in this life.

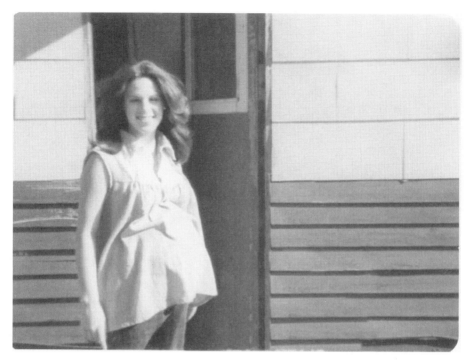

Laura pregnant with Arica, 1977

CHAPTER 4

The Gift of Imperfection

Many years had passed since my first tentative steps into parenthood, and I was in the middle of enjoying a new phase of life: grandparenthood. Being a grandparent is the abundant life on steroids. There is simply nothing like it. If God is my father, then He loves my children with the love of a grandparent: a love that grows and grows. With each new grandchild, my heart rejoices, and I love being included in my daughters' pregnancies.

As I sat in the ultrasound room with my daughter Mary, awaiting a peek at grandchild number seven, I took in my surroundings, immersed in a deep sense that I had been here before. The room was unremarkable, like most hospital rooms. There was Mary, reclining on the bed, waiting for the nurse to do her ultrasound. There was the ultrasound machine, giving off its eerie glow in the dim light. A nondescript, mass-produced painting hung on the wall. I sat in the token guest chair, pushed into the corner. I had been to lots of ultrasounds and doctors' appointments, even at this hospital, but there was something different about this one. Then, as the nurse squirted the gel onto Mary's stomach, it dawned on me. It wasn't déjà vu. I *had* been here before—in this exact room—twenty-three years before.

The younger version of me was here, alone, as the nurse squeezed the cold gel on my belly. I was so excited—the first look at my new baby. As with my other pregnancies, I knew there would be something magical in hearing my baby's heartbeat for the first time.

The nurse moved the probe around on my belly, and I couldn't help but smile in anticipation.

Any minute now, I thought. *Any minute….* Then suddenly I could see the sac. It was peanut shaped, not round like my others had been, yet I believed it was still beautiful.

After a few more moments, the nurse turned off the ultrasound machine, walked to the door, and said, "The doctor will be with you shortly."

Wait. What? Why hadn't she let me hear the heartbeat? I lay there in the dark, the paper on the bed crackling as I shifted my weight.

The doctor walked in with somber steps. "We were unable to find the heartbeat," he said. He went on to explain that I had what was called a blighted ovum, or anembryonic pregnancy. A blighted ovum occurs when a sperm and egg meet and attach to the uterine wall, but there is no life. It usually happens so early in pregnancy that a woman does not yet know she is pregnant. Cells form the pregnancy sac but not the embryo, and the placenta can continue to grow for a short time, which sustains a rise in pregnancy hormones even though there is no baby. Normally, a woman's body would eventually miscarry, but mine hadn't.

"Laura, you've lost your baby." He stared at me meaningfully. "There's no life inside the sac, and the sac itself is misshaped."

I just stared back. Honestly, I didn't believe him. I believed *he believed* what he was saying, but I had miscarried before and knew what it was to lose a baby. My body hadn't miscarried this time, so I still had hope. I just knew my baby was alive.

"We are going to schedule you for a D&C."

"No. I'm not going to do that."

"You've lost the baby. You have to do this for your health."

"No. I still have the baby. As long as there is life in my womb, I am not aborting."

"This isn't an abortion; it's a D&C." He was clearly annoyed.

"Well, it's the same procedure, and it takes life out. If this baby does not pass naturally with miscarriage, I'm not forcing it."

"You need to see a psychiatrist," he said, none too nicely.

I thanked the medical staff and left the room. Then I made a follow-up prenatal appointment with the front desk. As I exited the hospital, I pushed open the door and looked up to the sky and said boldly, "God, you raised Lazarus from the dead! Breathe life into my baby!" In my heart I recited Genesis 2:7 KJV, "And the Lord God formed man of the dust of the ground, and breathed into his nostrils the breath of life; and man became a living soul." I went home thanking God for my child. Looking back on it, I'm a little surprised at my audacity in telling God what to do. But I suppose I would have done the same with my earthly father, and God is my heavenly Father.

Over the next four weeks, I continued to have doctors' appointments. Though my pregnancy hormones continued to rise, they still could not find a heartbeat. The doctor, officially put out with me, persistently advocated for counseling and a D&C. With each successive appointment, the tension grew. The staff seemed convinced I would either succumb to infection any day or finally exhibit the symptoms of miscarriage. From the outside, I probably did seem crazy. Even my friend gently suggested that I was just being stubborn and should listen to the doctor's advice. It wasn't that I inherently mistrusted doctors or refused to accept the reality of miscarriage or stillbirth. I had experienced it. I know it happens to many women, and I don't want to lessen their pain or cast judgment on their unique situations. But even back then I maintained that God was the giver of life and that if this baby was not supposed to live, then I would miscarry. This conviction allowed me to persist week after week, grimace after grimace, and face a doctor who thought I was being irresponsible by continuing my pregnancy.

Then one day, there it was. Loud and clear. I heard my baby's heartbeat for the first time. It was music to my ears.

The doctor looked at me and said blandly, "I guess you were right."

"I know," I said, smiling triumphantly.

"We call that a 'medical miracle.' Make your next appointment," he said after casually shrugging his shoulders.

The shoulder shrug spoke volumes. I have been in many appointments with women who have high-risk pregnancies, and doctors are typically excited when there is good news about the pregnancy. It was strange to have my doctor treat this incredible news so nonchalantly. My mother had taught me to let nothing steal my joy, so I was determined nothing would, not even this doctor's indifference.

Months passed, and I enjoyed a normal pregnancy. Around my seventh month, however, the ultrasound alarmed the doctor again. My baby girl's head was too large and her femurs too short. They suspected dwarfism or another birth defect. My first response was, "That's okay. I can love a small person."

I was advised that I would need to validate the findings with a specialist at Alta Bates hospital to more accurately decide if I wanted to continue the pregnancy.

Continue the pregnancy? Had they forgotten I was the woman who prevailed with a pregnancy that lacked a heartbeat for weeks?

Now *they* were the crazy ones.

Women who 'choose' to have a child with Down syndrome are increasingly viewed by society as 'irresponsible.' This undermines the social position of people with Down syndrome and their families in society even more.

At the risk of sounding like an alarmist, I believe this is one way our society has allowed for an attack on the disabled. Anecdotal and academic research suggests that parents are often pressured to abort a child diagnosed with a birth defect, especially Down syndrome.[12,13] Many women have testified that, when given the diagnosis of Down syndrome, they were led to believe that it would be an almost certain outcome of poor quality of life for both the child and the family. These women were not given resources to see what life with a child with Down syndrome has been like for others; they were given very little hope at all, and abortion seemed to be the only option moving forward. In the United Kingdom, medical clinics have been known to hand out testing and termination flyers in tandem. Some women were told their marriages would certainly fail or that their older children would suffer if they continued the pregnancy. Others were offered the next available termination slot without being given the options of counseling or time to take in the news.

One woman said she was told of the next available termination opening *at every appointment* and finally had to note in her chart not to ask her again. There are even cases of doctors refusing to continue care for the woman if she rejected an abortion.[14] Further, one Down syndrome advocacy group states, "Women who 'choose' to have a child with Down syndrome are increasingly viewed by society as 'irresponsible.' This undermines the social position of people with Down syndrome and their families in society even more."[15]

I realize that numbers can often be misused on both sides of this argument, but if you will humor me, let me throw a few out here.

In 2016, 90 percent of people in the United Kingdom who found out their baby had Down syndrome chose abortion.[16] In Denmark, 98 percent of prenatal diagnoses of Down syndrome ended in abortion in 2015. That might seem impossibly high, but Iceland has them beat. According to numbers given in Icelandic parliament, beginning in 2008 and continuing to the present, of pregnancies diagnosed with Down syndrome, 100 percent have been terminated. I'll let that sink in. *All* of the babies diagnosed in utero as having Down syndrome have been aborted for the last *nine* years. And while testing is not compulsory, the report also stated that abstaining from testing is rare.[17]

Finally, according to statistics reviewed by Dr. Brian Skotko, a pediatric geneticist at Children's Hospital Boston, based on voluntary data, it is estimated that 92 percent of women in the United States who receive a prenatal Down syndrome diagnosis choose to have an abortion. Skotko goes further to state,

> *I am concerned about mothers making that informed decision. Are they making it on facts and up-to-date information? Research suggests not, and that mothers get inaccurate, incomplete and sometimes offensive information.*[18]

Some argue that terminating pregnancies of the possibly disabled is the only humane thing to do. They also argue—at times behind closed doors—that it prevents an unnecessary drain on society. Long an advocate for the disabled, Dr. Adrienne Asch and her colleague, Dr. David Wasserman, address this claim in the American Medical Association's *Journal of Ethics*:

> *While it may be reasonable to treat the incidence of disability among existing people as, in part, a public health*

problem, it is problematic to treat the existence of future people with disabilities that way. A policy of prevention-by-screening appears to reflect the judgment that lives with disabilities are so burdensome to the disabled child, her family, and society that their avoidance is a health care priority—a judgment that exaggerates and misattributes many or most of the difficulties associated with disability.

We believe the principal difficulties faced by people with disabilities and their families are caused or exacerbated by discriminatory attitudes and practices that are potentially remediable by social, legal, and institutional change—in much the same way that many of the difficulties associated with being African American or female in America have been ameliorated. A policy that promotes selection against embryos and fetuses with disabling traits conveys the strong impression that the problem is the disability itself rather than the society that could do so much more to welcome and include all its members.[19]

Hayley Goleniowska is a mother in Britain who was encouraged to have an abortion when testing revealed she was at a high risk for having a baby with Down syndrome. Despite the pressure, she continued her pregnancy and now advocates for those with Down syndrome on behalf of her beautiful daughter, whom she says has hugely benefited their entire family and shattered any "outdated preconception" of what life with a child with Down syndrome is like. She strongly believes that living with the differently abled is an enriching experience.

When discussing the argument that late-term abortion is a humane choice for those pregnancies deemed "not compatible with life," she notes that a parliamentary study shows that a number of children aborted under these pretenses have mild to moderate developmental delays, such as Down Syndrome, and superficial problems, such as cleft palate and club foot. That these conditions are classified as "not compatible with life" is alarming, and, as she puts it, "an uncomfortable truth if ever I stumbled across one."[20]

The problem is only getting worse. With new Noninvasive Prenatal Testing (NIPT) being introduced, many fear the abortion rates of those identified with disabilities will increase. And who is to say they will stop with Down syndrome? Will a target IQ be introduced? What about other genetic abnormalities? What about gender? In many parts of the world, being a female cannot only be a disadvantage, it can be a cause for suffering. Do we, then, support abortions based on genetic testing to spare females from the trials they may face? Where does it end?

Pondering these questions and our society's view of the disabled, I arrived at Alta Bates, a premier hospital in Northern California known for its work with pregnancy abnormalities. Normally, to test for abnormalities and genetic disorders, one would undergo an amniocentesis. This is a process in which a hollow needle is inserted into the uterus to extract a sample of amniotic fluid. The medical staff felt that this procedure was too dangerous for me at my late stage of pregnancy and might send me into pre-term labor, so they performed an ultrasound and ruled out dwarfism.

"There is more. You have a lot of excess fluid, and this indicates there will be brain damage. We can't tell how severe, because we can't perform the amniocentesis. You will just have to wait until the birth."

I could do that. I wasn't stunned. Everything about this pregnancy had been breathtakingly beautiful to me, and I knew it would continue to be even if this news wasn't. I had seen God's hand in this pregnancy, and I had full confidence in His handling of the situation. I prayed fervently that God would make her healthy, but I also knew that whatever He chose to do, He had chosen me to be her mother.

My daughter was born six and a half weeks premature. As confirmed, she was not a dwarf—in fact, she is my tallest child. She had no brain damage. She did suffer from respiratory distress syndrome (RDS) related to her premature birth, for which she needed extra oxygen to help her breathing. I remember staring at her caved-in chest. The doctor told me my daughter may not live through her first night, and I just smiled—this baby had already lived through so much. Once she was released from the NICU, I took this glorious girl—my hope held out for—home.

And now here I sat with Mary during her ultrasound, in the same room I had been in when they told me my pregnancy was over. Mary could not have understood the emotion going through me at the time, thinking about my previous experience in this place. She didn't know that she, too, had been here before. She was the blighted ovum, the baby who wasn't supposed to be. There she was, healthy and happy, looking at an image of her own beautiful baby.

I couldn't contain it. I had to tell her. Though she knows the story of her birth, she had no idea we were in the same room where it all started. She found it, well, *weird*, but she said she wasn't totally surprised. She had a feeling about me being at this appointment, like there was something special about it. Her appointment that day ended in a high-five, much different than mine had twenty-three years earlier.

Later that day she reminded me of what she says in every Mother's Day card: "Thank you, Mom. Thank you for giving me life and not listening to the doctors. Thank you for going with your gut and trusting God. If you hadn't, I wouldn't be here. I know I have a purpose. I know I am supposed to be here. Thank you for letting me be."

"God gave you life," I reminded her.

"Yes, but *you* listened to God."

What would I do without my Mary? Mary brings gentle peace wherever she goes. She is the calm in my storm. Whenever I'm feeling hyper or anxious, all she has to do is say, "Mom, how are you?" and I calm right down. She is my fifth and final child, and she has made all of our lives so full. Few people know or understand what a miracle she is.

But she almost wasn't here.

How many children are not here, because prenatal testing showed there could be abnormalities? There is no way to know how many of those tests were actually false positives like my own, but I know plenty of people who chose life anyway, only to have children without disabilities. A 2014 study by a California-based prenatal screening company found that 6.2 percent of women who were told screening indicated their baby was at a high risk for a chromosomal condition chose to abort *without getting any further testing.*[21]

And what of those who chose life and their child *does* have disabilities? Cultural norms and society's expectations of parents aside, if parents of disabled children could be completely honest, how many of them would say they wished their child had never been born? That is not to say that raising a child with disabilities is not impossibly hard at times. I realize it can be terribly difficult and lonely, and I have such admiration for parents who do it well. But given the choice, would they do it all over again? The parents I know would say a resounding, "Yes!"

Parents who have children with Down syndrome often say that those children have helped them see the world through completely new and wonderful eyes. That child has changed their family's life for the better. Raising a child with Down syndrome is a gift, and their siblings agree. According to British actress Sally Phillips, regarding life with her son with Down syndrome, "I was told it was a tragedy and actually it's a comedy. It's like a sitcom where something appears to go wrong but there's nothing bad at the end of it."[22]

My friends Tony and Lori know first-hand what it is to walk this road. Told when Lori was five months pregnant that soft markers indicated their third child had a high likelihood of Down syndrome, the couple were stunned. They had imagined what the future of their family would look like, and this was not it. Lori found it hard to bond with her baby in utero, because she just didn't fit the image she had created in her mind. She posted Psalm 139 on her mirror and kept repeating it to herself: *For you created my inmost being; you knit me together in my mother's womb. I praise you because I am fearfully and wonderfully made....All the days ordained for me were written in your book before one of them came to be.*[23]

Tony took a different approach. In college, he had worked with the cognitively disabled. Their situation was dire—stuck in a basement all day with very little quality of life. He didn't know what to expect for his own child, but he wanted to strategize and prepare. He went to the library and checked out every relevant book he could. What he found in those textbooks and brought home to Lori corroborated her worst fears. Page after page dwelt on the likely complications their daughter would face, from heart defects to poor dental formation. There was no silver lining, only pain.

Yet, as strong believers in the sanctity of life, the couple chose to continue their pregnancy. When their daughter was born, blue and in distress, all of Lori's hesitation vanished. She immediately felt the bond and knew she would do anything to fight for her baby. With the help of an incredible NICU, their daughter thrived. They named her Leilani Joy, little knowing how true the name would prove to be.

What all those scary textbooks and articles failed to mention were the upsides. They didn't tell them that Leilani would love big, enthusiastically greeting them with hugs every time she sees them or that she would be the most avid sports fanatic and athletically driven in their family. They didn't tell them that she would be reading before she ever started kindergarten or be the frequent reason the whole family would dance in the car. The research didn't foretell the way Leilani would help her siblings become even more responsible and compassionate, nor the profound effect she would have on her community and the way it perceived disability. In short, none of their research told them all the beautiful things they would miss if Leilani hadn't joined their lives.

"It was really unrealistic, looking back on it. If we were to anticipate all that was going to go wrong in our own bodies from the very beginning, we would be terrified. No one can live like that, and we aren't asked to," Lori says.

Tony agrees: "Trying to figure out how to fix everything before it happens doesn't work. You would be completely overwhelmed with things that might not ever even be an issue. You just have to let life run its course and deal with things as they come up."

It was frustrating for them that the larger medical community only portrayed all the negative possibilities. In both blatant and subversive ways, it became clear to them that there is a strong bias to terminate pregnancies where disability is suspected.

Sadly, this attack on the disabled is not new. Margaret Sanger, the founder of the nation's leading abortion provider, was actively involved in eugenics, the belief that actions must be taken to control the reproduction, usually through forced sterilization, of the segments of society the elite found undesirable. Depending on whom you spoke to, *undesirable* often referred to anyone who possessed the following characteristics: poor, non-white, physically or mentally disabled. When the Nazis later took a page from the playbook of Sanger and her eugenics colleagues, with whom they shared personal relationships, they infamously added *non-Arian*.

Sanger prominently believed in and crusaded toward achieving a society without the "unfit and mentally ill." In her book, *The Pivot of Civilization*, she argues:

The emergency problem of segregation and sterilization must be faced immediately. Every feeble-minded girl or woman of the hereditary type, especially of the moron class, should be segregated during the reproductive period. Otherwise, she is almost certain to bear imbecile children, who in turn are just as certain to breed other defectives. The male defectives are no less dangerous. Segregation carried out for one or two generations would give us only partial control of the problem. Moreover, when we realize that each feeble-minded person is a potential source of an endless progeny of defect, we prefer the policy of immediate sterilization, of making sure that parenthood is absolutely prohibited to the feeble-minded....

The lack of balance between the birth-rate of the "unfit" and the "fit," admittedly the greatest present menace to the civilization, can never be rectified by the inauguration of a cradle competition between these two classes. The example of the inferior classes, the fertility of the feeble-minded, the mentally defective, the poverty-stricken, should not be held up for emulation to the mentally and physically fit, and therefore less fertile, parents of the educated and well-to-do classes. On the contrary, the most urgent problem today is how to limit and discourage the over-fertility of the mentally and physically defective. Possibly drastic and Spartan methods may be forced upon American society if it continues complacently to encourage the chance and chaotic breeding that has resulted from our stupid, cruel sentimentalism.[24]

She further states in *Woman and the New Race:*

> *Birth control itself, often denounced as a violation of*
> *natural law, is nothing more or less than the facilitation of*
> *the process of weeding out the unfit, of preventing the birth of*
> *defectives or of those who will become defectives.*[25]

While many in the pro-choice movement are vocal about the
rights and treatment of the disabled and quick to defend anyone
who has been perceived to be discriminated against on the basis of
disability—as they certainly should be—they are actually complicit in
what some have called a genocide of the disabled population.[26] Hayley
Goleniowska has this to say about the hypocrisy of the culture:

> *In the West we pride ourselves on our equality laws, those*
> *that give each individual the same rights, whatever their*
> *gender, ethnicity, sexuality or disability. Yet we are shouting*
> *loud and clear to adults with disabilities that they are worth*
> *a little bit less with our abortion laws, and very few of us are*
> *questioning that.*[27]

That the founder of an organization that is the leading provider
of abortions in the United States championed the eradication of
the disabled should not come as a surprise. Her organization was
responsible for 323,999 abortions in one year alone. And that was
strictly surgical abortions performed in the 2014–2015 fiscal year,
according to their annual report. It does not count the babies aborted

through emergency contraception and other abortive drugs, such as RU-486 and ella. If you factor those numbers in, the number is well over 1.5 million lives lost in a single year to one "women's health" organization.[28]

Because of privacy laws and the sensitivity around the issue of abortion, it is unlikely that the United States will ever capture the data that will tell us accurately how many of those abortions were identified as "possibly disabled." And while we know a percentage of those abortions are simply a form of birth control to these women, one of the main reasons this organization and other pro-abortion groups claim abortion is necessary is the elimination of babies with disabilities or birth defects. They may pass it off as concern for the quality of life for the child, but the way they approach the issue and the information they provide parents makes clear that their idea of life with a disabled person does not match the reality of such for most people. Regardless, the result is the same: Thousands, if not hundreds of thousands, of babies are aborted every year based solely on the fact that they might have genetic defects. The abortion industry, and those who participate, are taking steps toward a disability-free society. It would make Margaret Sanger proud.

If we want to fight the loss of life to abortion, we must also fight the stigma of cognitive disability, as well as find ways to support families traveling this road. How do we do this? Lori, Tony, and other parents who have children with disabilities have a few suggestions:

- Be proactive about showing those with disabilities in our advertisements and promotions.

- Include those with genetic disabilities in the functions of our church so that church members see that community is built and made beautiful by all sorts of people.
- Share inspiring stories on our social media platforms.
- Follow the lead of Joel Osteen and implement programs like Champions Club[29] in our churches to minister to families living with disabilities, or throw a Night to Shine prom night for students with disabilities.[30] The pro-choice movement likes to claim that the church cares little for these children once they are born, but churches across the nation have shown the opposite is true by initiating these types of ministries.
- Look for ways to grow in welcoming families with disabilities into our churches. A very small percentage of families who have members with disabilities actually attend church because it is so difficult. Establish areas where those with differing needs can fully engage in the worship experience.
- Poll parents to see what sorts of things would be helpful for their family's worship experience, and create awareness and sensitivity among church members.
- Do not forget good old-fashioned TLC. If a family has a child with a disability, let the world see the church surrounding them and helping them along each step of the way.
- Offer to babysit so parents can have time for the paramount responsibility of maintaining a good marriage.
- Encourage and facilitate, if possible, their attendance to conferences where they can gather valuable information and support and be with other families who understand.

- Raise any low expectations of the cognitively disabled, for they are capable of far more than society believes. Just look at Karen Gaffney, the American woman with Down syndrome who swam the English Channel!

Lori stresses that is important to let expectant parents process the news in the best way for them:

> *Whatever you are feeling about the prospect of raising a child with a disability, that's okay. Process it. But don't let fear of the unknown prevent you from the joy this child will bring. The hope and the joy you get from raising a child with Down syndrome far outweighs the fear. You have so much more to lose by aborting your child than you do by keeping her. Abortion may seem like an easy out, but it will bring far more pain than it will peace.*

When people see happy, functioning families that include someone with a cognitive disability, social perceptions will begin to shift. When expectant parents have had a chance to observe what life is really like with a child with a disability, talk with parents who have walked that road, and see that they will not be alone, my hope is that they will not feel devastated when they hear the news that their child might be disabled. My dream is that they will sit there, in that room with the eerie glow of the ultrasound and the non-descript, mass-produced painting on the wall, and they will find the strength and the courage to continue with a new life.

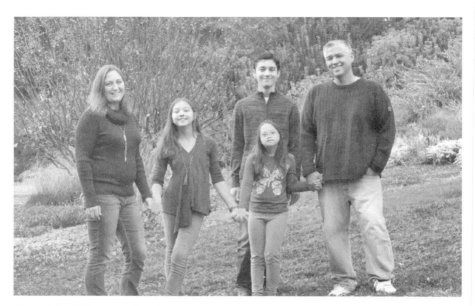

Tony & Lori Tiemann Family

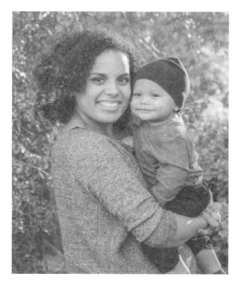

Mary & Malachi
Photography by SuzetteAllen.com

CHAPTER 5

Beauty for Ashes

As Pearl cradled her newborn baby boy and looked at the soft features of his face, her heart sang. He was perfection. The tiny nose, the grasping fingers…it was almost too much beauty to handle.

This child. This was her beauty born out of piles of long-buried ash. This was something she had done right. This was who she was living for now. She had been wrong about so many things in her life, but not this. This choice had given her power. Power to start a life, even now, for both of them. Her baby boy was all that mattered.

She had named him Adar, meaning *prince,* and he was royalty to her. "Twinkle, Twinkle" seemed a fitting song for a little prince, so she sang softly to him as she let the awe of this new life settle over her.

But her reverie was interrupted by incessant questions: What was she going to do? How would she provide for him? Could she be both father and mother to this child? Would she eventually tell her son about her past and…*him?*

Her eyes began to well up with tears as she looked at Adar in all his slumbering beauty. The sensation was different than it had been a few years earlier, when the tears hurt so badly as they fell across the gash on her face, courtesy of her pimp and a clothing iron that happened to be within his reach. He rightly suspected that she had been stashing money, preparing for escape. He needed to remind her that she had already been his property for three years and that there was no way out of her sex-trafficked life. Much like her pain, she hid the horrific details of this story the day we met.

The sun shining through the trees made a mosaic on the floor of the Alpha Pregnancy Clinic as I completed one of my regular shifts as a volunteer advocate. Hearing the familiar *swoosh* of the front door, I looked up and watched a young woman walk in. She was beautiful—absolutely stunning. Yet under her striking features, something gave me the feeling she had been hurt deeply in her past. It was clear she was second-guessing her decision to walk through that door.

At first, she was guarded and demure. We sat together on a couch in one of the consulting rooms. I could tell she was anxious, so I did what I often do with the women who come to see us: I told her to take a minute to breathe. I counted to five mentally, and I could visibly see her begin to relax. She was hesitant to speak. My mom had once told me that sharing my pregnancy story always broke the ice with the young women she ministered to in the Billings Alpha Pregnancy Clinic, so I commenced sharing my story and pregnancy journeys. The walls in which she had protectively enclosed herself began to crumble.

Pearl's story is tragic but beautiful. Tragic because of what she endured. Beautiful because she chose zoe—she chose life within the aftereffects of trauma and deeply-rooted pain. I met her before she had made that choice to bring life into this messed up, crazy world that she had so far survived with little to no support.

A few years free from being a sex slave and desperately trying to get her life together, she found out she was pregnant. She was on her way to the library one day when she noticed the Alpha Pregnancy Clinic was advertising free pregnancy tests and ultrasounds, and that's when she came in. Alone and unsure of herself, she was prepared to face strangers who would question who she was and how she had arrived at this point in her life. Instead, she told me later that what greeted her at the door was the overwhelming feeling of, "We're here for you. We are *so* here for you."

"Nothing was scripted," she told me as our friendship developed. "I could tell everything was from the heart. The staff and volunteers at the Alpha Pregnancy Clinic let me cry and be real with what I felt, but *then they got excited!* It gave me permission to be excited! I wanted to be excited, but had felt like I couldn't be."

Something just clicked, and from that very first meeting, we formed a special connection. She felt like one of my daughters. I'll never forget the expression on her face as she looked at the baby models and saw what her baby looked like at that early, first trimester stage. She carefully touched the cherry-sized replica, with its little webbed fingers and toes. Her smile was the smile of a woman in love.

Pearl came to the center frequently, and we practiced the basics of baby care. We discussed how to hold a baby gently and position him for nursing or bottle-feeding. We practiced washing an infant correctly—in a small basin with a washcloth, ensuring he was held safely above water at all times. We went over swaddling tightly to help him sleep, as well as other soothing techniques like rocking and singing. We examined the importance of stepping away from the baby and finding a safe, quiet place if the crying became too much and she felt herself getting angry, frustrated, or tempted to shake him to make him be quiet. We watched videos together that explained what was happening with her body and ways to continue a healthy pregnancy and prepare her home for the safe arrival of a baby. We talked about resources available to her and her baby once he was born, as well as materials that could help her prepare, like the books *What to Expect When You're Expecting* by Heidi Murkoff and Sharon Mazel, and *The Wonder Within You: Celebrating Your Baby's Journey from Conception to Birth* by Carey Wickersham.

There was laughter and there were tears, but most of all there was relationship, and Pearl knew she was not alone.

I was struck by the way she craved advice. Anything she could do to help the life inside her, she did. She was teachable. And she was so brave. It would take a large quantity of both skills to manage her future with a newborn child as a single parent—that I knew well from my own experience—yet I also knew that not only was she going to be okay, she was going to do it well.

I often hear the argument that abortion spares a child from a difficult life. I have even heard the argument that *not* choosing abortion is selfish on the part of the mother, should she expect difficulty for her child. Why wouldn't a mother spare her child the suffering? But I would ask: Is all difficulty bad? Do difficulties in life not provide us the opportunity to grow stronger and more useful, like a clay pot exposed to fire in a kiln? Is the possibility of hardship in a child's life justification for snuffing out that life altogether?

And by what and whose standards do we judge what a "good" life is?

Economic stability? While we all want to be economically sound, I would wager that there are many children in the developing world whose standard of living pales in comparison to that of those in the United States, but still believe it is a life worth living. Even within affluent societies, there are and always have been those who enjoy a tremendous satisfaction in a life outside the status quo of material wealth. Perhaps our culture needs to take a closer look at what level of economic status is needed for true happiness.

Single-parent household? I know all about that. It's hard. It's really, really hard. But it is doable. Children want your love. If you give them that, there is so much of the other "stuff" society says they need that they are perfectly happy to do without. When they were growing up, my kids would sometimes describe our family as poor, because of our financial situation. I always reminded them that we were rich in love. We had God, and we had each other.

Stability in the home? There are many heartbreaking situations in our world. I know this. I do not pretend to have the answer for all of them or hope to wave some magic wand of words and assume that it will dissolve all the truly difficult and overwhelming things people face. I do not want anyone reading this book to think I am trivializing the devastating positions in which some women find themselves. But might I gently encourage you to encourage women: What better time for action than now? If a woman finds herself in a situation that is untenable and unsafe for a baby, it is likely untenable and unsafe for her. The baby's life is not expendable; neither is hers. Get out. Do everything in your power to help her get out. Perhaps having this new life inside her will be the impetus she needs to finally have the courage to break free. If a woman is in an abusive relationship in which she fears her partner will abuse the child, yet will not consent to an adoption, she has options to protect her child that do not have to include abortion. Both adoption agencies and departments of family services can help women navigate these complex situations in a way that lets both her and her child survive.

Pearl understood difficulty. Over time, she opened up about her story. There had been no one to sing lullabies to her twenty-four years earlier when she lay as a newborn in a tiny hospital bed. Abandoned by her drug-addicted mother, three days passed before a great aunt claimed her and agreed to take her home.

Pearl was grateful to Great Aunt Tee for taking her in—truly—but she dubbed her aunt's house "home" in the loosest sense of the word. She always felt like an outsider, mostly due to her cousins, Aunt Tee's "real" kids, who constantly reminded her that she was trespassing by living with their family. The situation and resentment only grew worse when her aunt took charge of Pearl's two younger brothers as well.

Aunt Tee, fatiguing with age and over-extended with a houseful of kids to care for, showed little affection for Pearl. There was an expectation of behavior and a long list of prohibitions, but what was sorely lacking was the mutual trust and respect between caregiver and child that research shows is integral for effective discipline and maturity of the child.[31] If Pearl kept to herself and didn't cause trouble with Aunt Tee or her cousins, she was left alone. So, detached she continued, hiding her life away. She never sought advice, and it was never offered. The lack of involvement in her life by an adult meant she wasn't given chances to make mistakes within a controlled environment and learn from them while consequences were small, before making much larger ones in the world where the repercussions were life-altering.

At age eighteen, Pearl left home. Now she was on her own and trying to survive. There were so many decisions! Before long, she had new friends who gave her advice *and* affection. She felt like she was known and cared for, not just a dependent in need of food and shelter. Because of this, their influence meant so much more than the lectures from Aunt Tee. They fed her ego, and the newfound control of being on her own was liberating. Now was her chance to be the torchbearer to light the way for her own life. But with no guidance, instead of shining light on the path to her future, she set it ablaze. Some of her friends introduced her to a man who promised to help her pay her bills. He was charming. He flattered her meager self-worth. She went along. At the time, she didn't realize the steep price that would be exacted by her naiveté.

She endured the searing pain of being sex-trafficked for three years. Not long after the iron-to-the-face incident, having convinced her pimp she needed to stop at a gas station to use the restroom, she made her move. She had tried to stop crying, to be quiet as she hid beneath the cash register of the sympathetic store clerk. But the salt from the tears stung her wound, and she winced. She must remain silent. *He* was there. *He* was looking for her. *He* was shouting at the clerk. She was his, and he would find her and take her back. How long had she waited there? She couldn't remember. The clerk had locked up and told her to wait and make sure the pimp was gone. Then he called the police.

When the police arrived, she didn't want to press charges, because she never wanted to see her captor again. She wanted to run away to the big city, to hide in its anonymity. She asked the police just to let her be, and she began to make her way on foot from the isolated gas station to the bus station in the next town. On that long, lonely road, she came across a construction crew.

To her, the expressions on their faces after one look at her battered, disheveled appearance, told her they understood that her life had not been kind. They seemed to want to help.

Someone wanted to help her? It was such a foreign concept.

They comforted her, and she felt the faint beginnings of trust. She gratefully accepted a ride to the bus station. But...

The drive included a detour to the house of one of the men. When they got there, more men were waiting. Instead of finding help, she was gang-raped by ten men. Her fragile trust was crushed yet again.

Left on her own, bruised and broken, she wrapped herself in her shame and somehow made it into the city.

Eventually, she ended up back at Aunt Tee's, but there was no solace there. No one could know she had been sex-trafficked, least of all Tee. In a moment of weakness, she began to tell her story to a cousin, but instead of compassion and comfort, she was met with utter disgust and disdain. The shame and horror of her past was a burden she believed she must bear on her own. So, she did. And as

Chapter 5

far as her family is concerned, so she does to this day. They couldn't accept the imperfect, broken fragments of her; they only wanted a whole and unblemished facade.

Despite insurmountable odds, Pearl pieced her life back together. Things were going well. She was working as a medical caregiver and pursuing a license as a certified nurse's assistant. She thought she even found love. But "love" can be fickle, and things changed when she discovered she was pregnant. Adar's father said he needed time to get used to the idea of being a parent, so she gave him space and told him to come back when he was ready to be in their lives. He never did. Instead, he began a relationship with a different woman who was already pregnant with another man's baby. The knife was double-edged: Not only did he choose that woman over Pearl, he chose another man's baby over his own. She was on her own *again*.

She could feel the flames starting to lick at the edges of her life. But this time, something was different. This time, there was a someone, and he—her precious child—was depending on her. Pearl knew from the start that the life she created was her responsibility. She had made a choice with her body, and this child was the result. She could not turn away from her duty to see this through. And though she wasn't sure how she would manage being a parent, she knew she would go down fighting anything or anyone who tried to harm him.

Even though she was scared, her determination led her to seek help at the Alpha Pregnancy Clinic, and that decision carried her healthily through her pregnancy to deliver her son. Six months after Adar was born, though she was still working in the medical field, pain became her reality again. A budding relationship with a friend failed, and she was kicked out of his relative's home, leaving her and Adar homeless. When they entered the homeless shelter, she was already struggling with postpartum depression and felt powerless as a mother. Adar became so ill he had to be rushed to the hospital, and when the doctor told her Adar had contracted tuberculosis at the shelter, she had never felt so low.

Devoting herself to Adar is what helped her cope. Her family hadn't shown her how to love. They never even said, "I love you." But she was determined it would be different for Adar. Through encouragement and practical help from her church, she fought for him and learned how to love in the process.

She had Adar, and Adar had her. Together they persisted, and together they were going to make a life. Today Adar is a happy, intelligent, thriving child. Do they still face difficulty? Yes. Is she still working through the pain of a traumatic past? Yes. As a person who has endured more than most of us, it may take Pearl a lifetime to reach the restoration that is possible for her. She hasn't "arrived," at least according to societal standards of success. She's not in a perfect place yet. But that isn't the point. The point is that she's pursuing wholeness—physical, emotional, and spiritual healing—so that she can give Adar the best of herself.

I am in no way trying to harp on the difficulties that Pearl has faced. She is an amazing mother. She is made of such tough stuff, and I am so proud of her. What I *am* trying to do is show you a real person, with real struggles, who still rejoices that she made the decision to keep her unplanned pregnancy.

If adversity in life is justification for death, what about those who had a happy, full childhood, but then trauma and affliction struck? Would it have been better for them to never have been born? If so, how would we foresee their fate and determine it was not a life worth living? If we were to be consistent, the person in question, of course, would have no say in the process. Their chance to live life would be determined wholly by others' interpretation of the risks.

Cannot the same logic be applied to children who may face adversity in childhood but go on to lead extraordinary lives? Would they say their benefit to society was moot because of their struggle?

When Helen Keller was nineteen months old, she was afflicted with an illness that left her both blind and deaf. Against all odds, she learned to read braille and communicate with the world around her. She went on to obtain an excellent education and became a driving force in the movement to improve treatment of and services for the disabled. She is given much credit for changing the way the world perceived disabled people. She authored several books, one of which is still in print in over fifty languages, and along with her teacher, was the subject of the award-winning play, *A Miracle Worker*. She is the hallmark of a person whose tenacity overcame adversity.

Considered one of the most brilliant cosmologists and theoretical physicists of all time, Stephen Hawking was diagnosed with Amyotrophic Lateral Sclerosis (ALS) prior to his twenty-first birthday. The disease robbed him of his mobility and speech, yet he has persevered. His work has had a tremendous effect on how the cosmic universe is understood.

When he was fifteen years old, Elie Wiesel, along with his family, was transported by the Nazis to Auschwitz concentration camp. The Nazi death camps claimed the lives of both his parents and a sister. After being liberated in 1945, Wiesel went on to author more than sixty books, including his acclaimed memoir, *Night.* For his work in exposing the atrocities that occurred during the Holocaust and preventing future human rights violations, Wiesel was awarded the Presidential Medal of Freedom, the U.S. Congressional Gold Medal, the National Humanities Medal, the Medal of Liberty, the 1986 Nobel Prize for Peace, and the rank of Grand-Croix in the French Legion of Honor.

Helen Keller, Stephen Hawking, and Elie Wiesel are only three among a plethora of people who have overcome adversity to impact our world. By the current argument that abortion saves children who will experience hardship or extreme suffering, these should have never been given life. What a travesty to our world.

And should you be tempted to think only famous people have made a difference, I would like to point out there are countless people who have overcome tremendous challenges and have quietly gone about their lives, making the world better for those in their spheres of influence. These people haven't received any public accolades, been published, or created name recognition for themselves. But you know them. My dear friend Derrick comes to mind. Shot in the neck by a drive-by shooter at age eighteen, he became a quadriplegic. Nonetheless, he received a college degree and married a beautiful woman with whom he has twins, a boy and a girl. He dedicates himself to helping people with disabilities find work. Derrick is one of the smartest and kindest overcomers I know. Several others have, no doubt, impacted your life. Imagine your life, and this world, without them. Perhaps *you* are one of them. If so, in the spirit of *It's a Wonderful Life*, imagine this world without you.

Adversity does not eradicate the impact of a life. And to be frank, annihilation does not either. The echoes of a life, no matter how brief or hidden, will be felt throughout eternity. My hope, though, is that each life be given a chance to carry its own torch, bright and clear, to its God-ordained finish line. Only heaven knows the Kellers, Hawkings, and Wiesels who have been kept from life in the name of mercy.

Wait, some might say. *What if Hitler, Stalin, or Pol Pot had been aborted? Wouldn't that have been better for society?* That's a tough one, I admit it. I do not fully understand the evil that drove those men and others like them to commit the atrocities that they did. In large part, they believed they could be gods, granting life and death. Just like Adam and Eve in the garden, when humanity assumes deity, things don't turn out well. Only God should grant life and death. But even knowing this, how can anyone know what future decisions a fetus will make? The only thing in our power is that *we* can choose to live a zoe life in such a way that it affects the world around us. We can do our best to overcome evil with goodness, and when it seems like the opposite is happening, we stand in love despite the evil. When we offer mercy, life flourishes.

Mercy, true mercy, is what allowed Pearl to continue with her pregnancy even when she was discouraged. Now with every milestone, Pearl rejoices that she brought this life into the world. Each time she sees Adar experience something she never got to do as a child, she feels like she has been given a gift. Seeing his face on

Christmas morning outshines all the images of the past. Though they are in a much better place now, her life can still be messy and hard, which means that at times her son's life is messy and hard. *But he has life.* She has given him that.

I care for all the women I've connected with at the Alpha Pregnancy Clinic, but I have a special place in my heart for Pearl. After Adar was born, she gave me an amazing gift: She asked me to be his godmother. What an honor! What a responsibility! Pearl makes it easy, though. I just sit back and watch the incredible job she is already doing and applaud her. I cherish the photos she texts me of his triumphs. When Adar was just three, he came in my door one day and recited the entire Lord's Prayer. Every time he comes to my house, he grabs the cross in the entryway. Holding it like a trophy, he proclaims how Jesus suffered because God loves us, and how He died on the cross for our sins. It's easy to imagine Adar impacting the world as an adult. Already he has impacted mine. This child is going places, and I'm so thrilled to be along for the ride.

I would love to tie up Pearl's story for you in a pretty little bow and show you a neatly wrapped package. My heart would rejoice to tell you everything is perfect for her now and all the pain is far, far behind her. But that isn't honest, and that isn't life. She still has pain. Sometimes her childhood attacks her. She will continue to have messy parts that need to be figured out. But what her life also has is Adar, and he is pure beauty. His life, and what lies before him, is full of potential. He basks in the glow of a devoted and loving mother who will and has sacrificed whatever she could for his good. Their life isn't perfect, but it is *life,* and it is beautiful.

CHAPTER 6

The Power of an Image

It's hard to measure the value of an image. Photography has the power to equalize, bear witness, and transport.

A solitary man stands in Tiananmen Square, his monochromatic white shirt and black pants in stark contrast to the army green of the four tanks that appear poised to run over him. I feel his resolute courage.

Naked, a screaming Vietnamese girl runs toward me on a road, flanked by other sobbing children doing the same. Behind her walk the soldiers, a billowing cloud of smoke and napalm at their backs. I can almost smell the burning flesh.

Forlorn, a mother sits staring off into the distance, her fingers resting by her mouth. Her children, hair cropped short, hide their faces behind her back. The lack of color does not hide the dirt and fatigue. I begin to understand the despair that was the Great Depression.

A girl stares at me from beneath a red headscarf. Her large, bright green eyes match the wall behind her and the patches of cloth showing through her torn garment. She is from another continent, culture, and time, yet in her haunting eyes I see myself. I see our common humanity.

All of us have seen images that have transformed us in some way or another. Images have the power to change society, to end war, to bring justice. They can drive us to action, and both encourage or horrify a nation. An entire generation of children encountered, perhaps for the first time, the stark reality of risk and death as they sat in their classrooms and watched the images of the heralded Space Shuttle Challenger exploding. A nation watched in collective horror and grief as an airplane ripped through the Twin Towers, smoke billowing. And we said a prayer of renewed determination and hope as we watched New York City firefighters raise a flag over the rubble.

I was so drawn to the beauty and importance of images that I became a photographer. I relish capturing moments that families can cherish long after their brains begin to grow fuzzy and wipe out the actual memories. When I do my annual photo shoots for children with special needs, their joy infects me, and I love that their beautiful spirits can be immortalized in a photograph. Most of all, I feel blessed that I can retain snatches of memories of my own children and grandchildren. On the rare occasion that my son is not deployed and all five of my children are together, I make it a point to take a family portrait—those faces are all that I hold dear. When I gaze at my family masterpiece, I am reminded about God's love for us, His children.

There have been many images that have shaped my life, but one of the most significant ones is the one my second daughter, Amanda, handed me one day as I pulled up into the driveway. She was so excited, she didn't even let me get out of the car.

"What's this?" I asked.

"Just open it," she said, eyes glittering.

It was a card thanking me for being a good mom and…an ultrasound. The picture of a perfect, beautiful baby. The world stood still. I stared at Amanda in disbelief. I know, I know. Is it really *that* exciting? It was a normal ultrasound of a human baby—I've seen hundreds.

But this was Amanda's ultrasound, and Amanda had been told she would never be able to hold such a picture of her own. In sheer elation I managed, "You're having a baby!"

Amanda not only had severe endometriosis, but she was also born with a blocked fallopian tube and a bicornuate uterus. *Bicornuate* literally means *two horns* in Latin, and in this condition, the uterus is heart-shaped and split in two, separated by a septum. Depending on the degree of separation, pregnancy is still possible, but often high risk. When Amanda was eighteen, she had surgery to degut the endometriosis, at which point her doctor said that the combination of her problems would make it impossible for her to conceive, let alone carry a pregnancy to term, and she would need to consider a surrogate. Yet, here I sat, holding a picture of my developing grandbaby—a little blip of a human being, full of potential. Holding that image felt like holding the sun; it was miraculous. My mother and I had fasted and prayed for nearly a decade for Amanda to one day have a child. This was the day our hope was fulfilled, and I have a picture to prove it.

Women are often denied the ability of seeing such pictures at abortion clinics. One young woman who visited the pregnancy resource center where I volunteer was moved to tears when we were preparing her ultrasound.

"Is that a monitor? You're going to let me see it?" she said. "The other clinic would not let me see it."

I can understand why. Seeing the image of a baby in utero can have a profound effect. To see the image and to hear the heartbeat—present on the twenty-first day in utero—powerfully changes our perspective. It becomes hard to ignore that a human is growing in there. One of the lies of abortion is that the fetus is devoid of individual humanity; it is an unnecessary clump of cells, less than an appendix. They insist on scientific terminology for the stages of development: *zygote, embryo, fetus.* This is a clever tactic because many people do not know that the literal translation of these words is *yoke, young one,* and *offspring.* If it isn't called a *baby,* surely it isn't one, right? To be clear, I have nothing against science. I only wish the pro-abortion camp would be consistent in their use of it, because science is clear on this: Individual, human life begins at conception. Personhood is extended to all.

This point was made clear by several medical specialists in their 1981 testimonies to the United States Senate Judiciary Subcommittee on Separation of Powers concerning this issue. Professor Hymie Gordon of Mayo Clinic gave his professional opinion, saying, "By all the criteria of modern molecular biology, life is present from the moment of conception." This was supported by the testimony of Dr. Alfred M. Bongiovanni, professor of pediatrics and obstetrics at the University of Pennsylvania:

> *I have learned from my earliest medical education that human life begins at the time of conception...I submit that human life is present throughout this entire sequence from conception to adulthood and that any interruption at any point throughout this time constitutes a termination of human life...I am no more prepared to say that these early stages [of development in the womb] represent an incomplete human being than I would be to say that the child prior to the dramatic effects of puberty...is not a human being. This is human life at every stage.*

Dr. Jerome LeJeune, the late professor of genetics at the University of Descartes in Paris, who discovered the chromosomal pattern of Down syndrome, added:

> *After fertilization has taken place a new human being has come into being...not a metaphysical contention, it is plain experimental evidence.... Each individual has a very neat beginning, at conception.*

Professor Micheline Matthews-Roth from Harvard University Medical School affirmed these views:

It is incorrect to say that biological data cannot be decisive... It is scientifically correct to say that an individual human life begins at conception... Our laws, one function of which is to help preserve the lives of our people, should be based on accurate scientific data.

And Dr. Watson A. Bowes from the University of Colorado Medical School[32] reinforced the belief that biological life begins at conception, stating:

The beginning of a single human life is from a biological point of view a simple and straightforward matter, the beginning is conception. This straightforward biological fact should not be distorted to serve sociological, political, or economic goals.

The abortion movement fights images and the use of ultrasound, and they fight them hard, almost as if they have something to hide. In an online video, one young woman tells of her abortion experience. Being a naturally curious person, following her abortion she asked to see the container that held the "product of her conception." Horrified, the clinic staff denied her and emphatically said, "You can't see that." Why wouldn't they let her see it? I have a friend whose doctor let her take her appendix home in a jar, yet we have been told a fetus is no different.

In the annual report of the nation's largest abortion provider, they state: "Thanks to our attorneys' work, we were also able to block a mandatory ultrasound law in North Carolina, which had no medical purpose and would have only served to shame women accessing basic health care."[33]

First, I question if abortion should be classified as "basic health care," and second, I don't know why women would be shamed when viewing an ultrasound if the fetus was, indeed, just a blob of tissue. Do women feel shame when they are shown an ultrasound of a cyst that is about to be removed? Now, please understand, I want no woman to feel shame. That isn't my point. In fact, I feel the abortion industry is putting women at greater risk for the trauma of shame and regret by withholding information. What I *am* saying is that clearly there is more going on in a woman's womb than the abortion industry would have us believe.

Truly, the interior of a woman's womb during pregnancy is a miracle. The fact that a baby's genetic makeup, including its sex, is complete at the moment of fertilization is astounding. But it just keeps getting more incredible. Dr. G. Donald Royster is a Reproductive-Endocrinologist and Infertility Specialist (REI), who also happens to be the doctor who cared for my third child, Amanda, during her remarkable pregnancy. Due to his work with fertility, he has more opportunity than most to observe the beginning stages of pregnancy. When asked about his view on fetal development, he had this to say:

> *To see the specialization of these cells going from a single*
> *cell, to eight cells, to hundreds of cells in just a few days, and*
> *from there developing into the separate parts of the fetus—*

that's amazing. Every day there is so much advancement of that fetal development and I'm definitely still in awe every step of the way.[34]

Dr. Royster also looks forward to what he affectionately and unofficially calls "the gummy bear stage":

At six to seven weeks you can make out the brain, head and the tail, but you can't really see any other structures. Just two weeks later, at about eight to nine weeks, you can see arm buds and leg buds. You can actually see the fetus moving, not just the heartbeat. And that's when it hits home, "This is a person." That's pretty amazing.

Amazing indeed. Embryos have been shown to turn away from light touch at seven and a half weeks, and brain waves have been measured as early as eight and a half weeks. According to the Endowment for Human Development (EHD):

Experts estimate the 10-week embryo possesses approximately 90% of the 4,500 body parts found in adults—including unique fingerprints. This means that approximately 4,000 permanent body parts are present just eight weeks after conception. Incredibly, this highly complex 10-week embryo weighs about 1/10th of an ounce and measures slightly less than 1¼ inches from head to rump.[35]

Clearly, just because something is small does not mean it is not complex or holds no value. The EHD notes further milestones of development:

- By eleven weeks, fetuses move their heads and jaws, sigh, stretch, and suck their thumbs. The number of heartbeats is close to exceeding ten million. Female fetuses already possess a uterus, ovaries, and reproductive cells. When I teach this in high schools, students are amazed to learn that a baby actually pees in the mother's womb at this stage.
- At twelve weeks, toenails and fingernails all begin to form and bones begin to harden.
- At thirteen weeks, a fetus has a fully formed nose and lips and is capable of intricate facial expressions.
- In the fourteenth week, the mouth and tongue contain taste buds, arms reach final proportion to body size, and the fetus is producing various hormones.
- At eighteen weeks, the formation of breathing passages is complete and the fetus releases stress hormones when poked with a sharp needle.
- By twenty-two weeks, the cochlea has reached adult size and the fetus begins responding to sound. The development of skin layers is also concluded. Some medical centers report survival rates as high as 40 percent for babies outside the womb at this stage.
- At twenty-six weeks, a baby can recognize its mother's voice and be startled by loud external noises, resulting in blinking, increased heart rate, movement, and swallowing; lungs are

producing the substance needed for breathing post birth.

• By twenty-eight weeks, a baby can smell and produce tears.

I have heard the argument that a fetus cannot feel pain, thus abortion is humane. However, scientific evidence is clear that a fetus can feel pain by twenty weeks, and some argue as early as eight weeks.[36] As Dr. Condic describes, "The neural circuitry responsible for the most primitive response to pain, the spinal reflex, is in place by 8 weeks of development. This is the earliest point at which the fetus experiences pain in any capacity." Dr. Condic goes on to explain that "a fetus responds just as humans at later stages of development respond; by with withdrawing from the painful stimulus." Knowing the unborn child feels pain early in pregnancy, Condic says the question is what to do with that information:

> *Imposing pain on any pain-capable living creature is cruelty. And ignoring the pain experienced by another human individual for any reason is barbaric. We don't need to know if a human fetus is self-reflective or even self-aware to afford it the same consideration we currently afford other pain-capable species. We simply have to decide whether we will choose to ignore the pain of the fetus or not.*

All of the many stages of fetal development highlight the sheer awesomeness that is the creation of a human being. No wonder the abortion movement tries to draw attention away from this miracle by discouraging the use of images. Women have testified that being educated about the scientific reality of what is occurring in their bodies helped inform their decision to choose life.[37] Conversely, women have lamented that, had they known the scientific facts of fetal development or been given a chance to see an ultrasound image of their baby, they would have chosen life instead of abortion.[38] One cannot say for certain what a woman will choose if given the ability to view her ultrasound, but I do know that providing ultrasounds to women with unplanned pregnancies through organizations such as Focus on the Family's Option Ultrasound has saved lives and is a straightforward way to help the cause for life. A picture may be worth a thousand words, but my reality is that a picture saves thousands of lives.

Seven months after Amanda showed me her ultrasound, sixteen of us gathered in a delivery room to witness the fruition of a dream dared hoped for. Yes, sixteen—my family doesn't do anything halfway. Unfortunately, her husband, Jeff, was not among the sixteen. Amanda had gone into labor early, and Jeff was still at his out-of-state school. Thanks to technology, however, we were able to establish a live internet connection so that he could be part of it. Dr. Royster, who had taken such good care of Amanda throughout her pregnancy, was scheduled to be on a family vacation in Hawaii, but he stopped by on his way to the airport to check on her and deliver a beautiful pink hat his wife had knitted for his littlest patient.

We were all giddy with excitement, and the room buzzed with our collective energy, punctuated with the sounds of Amanda's effort to give birth. After what seemed like an eternity, little Hartlee entered our world, perfect in every way.

But something was wrong. Blood was pooling on the floor.

Why was there so much blood? Why was the medical staff so intense?

"She's bleeding out," the doctor said. "Everyone but her mother, you need to get out—now!"

Stunned, family members made their way out of the room, slipping on Amanda's blood as they went. They scattered to the waiting room, where they sat in anxious silence, staring at the blood on their shoes and their red footprints in the hall. Her best friend, upon seeing her being wheeled down the hall, began to scream, "Please, God, don't take my best friend!" Jeff, sitting alone in a room in North Dakota, was in despair, wondering why his connection had cut out right after a flurry of activity began. We all prayed.

As the room cleared, the doctor said to me, "She needs surgery. I'm going to take care of Amanda, I need you to take care of *her*. Do you understand?"

He placed Hartlee in my arms and rushed Amanda out. The silence seemed strange in the wake of such chaos. Slowly and purposefully I began to snuggle skin-to-skin and sing to my new granddaughter. I knew it was important that she be welcomed into the world with peace and love. My feet were standing in my daughter's blood, but I knew I was holding a miracle and believed God was performing another miracle in the surgery room.

And He did.

After five days in the hospital, Amanda was released. Once assured she would never bear children, she has delivered three, and some of my favorite images are of Hartlee proudly holding the ultrasounds of her coming siblings.

Ultrasounds are some of the most important images out there, but there is one even more critical, and I can't really write a chapter on the value of images without mentioning it. In Genesis 1:27, we are told that God created human beings in His own image. We are His *eikons* (where we get our modern term *icon*), His likeness, His small representations. Theologian N.T. Wright puts it beautifully when he states that we are like angled mirrors, reflecting God's image and love to the world around us and reflecting creation's praise back to God.[39] That is a tremendous responsibility. As the church, we reflect God's love to a hurting world by choosing zoe and showing them how to do so as well. If the image of an unborn child has the power to effect change, how much more so a living, breathing representation of a God who desperately loves the world and wants to bring not just life, but a good, abundant life?

I heard a story recently of a young woman in her early twenties at a grocery checkout line. As she stood there with five children under the age of five and of various racial backgrounds, she could hear the couple behind her, one of whom was wearing a pro-life T-shirt, discussing her situation.

"Look at all those kids. She knows how they get here, right?"

"And it looks like they all have different fathers. Goodness."

"Oh, of course. She's using government assistance. Our tax dollars hard at work."

It should not have mattered to the couple how many children this woman had or how she was caring for them. While they may have questioned this woman's choices, they spoke about the children as if they were a burden, not a blessing. They should have applauded her for choosing life, if they truly were against abortion. They could have offered her encouragement or paid for her groceries. Instead they judged her and missed a chance to bless someone. Rather than speaking with love, they spoke the kind of words that might drive a woman to end her pregnancy. Though their reaction should have been different regardless, I think that couple would have found it interesting to know that the young woman did not give birth to any of those children. She was a foster mom, making great sacrifices at a young age to improve the lives of children who needed someone to love them. They could have learned much from her.

I truly believe that the unkind couple in the above story does not represent the majority of those in the pro-life movement. The people I know would never behave in such a way. However, this story does speak to the narrative—often inaccurate, but believed nonetheless— that the pro-life movement only cares about a baby before he or she is born. That is the image the world perceives. I know this isn't usually true, and the stories in these pages have shown the tangible ways we can and do demonstrate love for all life, both before and after birth. Yet, this is the pervasive impression our culture has of the pro-life movement. Hardly the reflection of God we desire.

We must take our role as image bearers seriously by combating this image with thoughtful action. First, it is imperative that we recognize the hypocrisy we might have in our own lives. How do we speak about those whom we've deemed to make irresponsible choices, or who are hard on their luck, or with whom we don't agree? Do we affirm their value beyond their ability to bring a life into the world or believe they deserve respect and compassion even though we may disapprove of their choices? There is no dignity without respect, and if we say all life has dignity, we must act accordingly. When we demonstrate care for *all* life, both before and after birth, we show our sincerity in our proclaimed intention to help bring God's kingdom to earth.

Donating our time and resources to support foster, adoptive, teen, or single parents is an excellent way to directly impact lives that others may have found unwanted. Whether by offering free babysitting or respite care, providing meals, donating resources with which parents can buy needed items, checking in on a regular basis to see if the families have any needs, or offering counseling or other services, putting our hand to the task of improving vulnerable lives or those saved from abortion will go a long way in showing our sincerity. We must realize our goal is not just about seeing a baby delivered but about building a family.

When we demonstrate care for *all* life, both before and after birth, we show our sincerity in our proclaimed intention to help bring God's kingdom to earth.

And our own families can be the most powerful images we have to show the world: They are a beacon on a hill. We must take a hard look at the way we portray family life to the world. As parents, there is a great temptation to seek solidarity and sympathy from others who are experiencing the not-so-glamorous side of parenting. I get it. I've been there. This need for camaraderie is not bad. However, the way I often see it played out in the media and on social networking sites can be detrimental to the way culture views children. The true blessing that having a child is gets lost somewhere in all the mess and fatigue. The highs of parenting are often overshadowed by the lows. Granted, the lows are entertaining in retrospect, but what develops is an underlying sense that children are a burden who steal from you all the things you used to love: your sleep, social life, sex life, body, clean house, finances…the list goes on. A crisp and beautiful picture has been traded for a worn and faded one. Why on earth would anyone on the fence about parenting sign up for *that*?

Often we don't think about the effect our words have, because *we* know the value and love that we have for our children and assume others inherently understand that unspoken piece. It is similar to how you can say something unkind about a member of your family, but if anyone else tries to do the same, you jump to your family's defense. What we don't realize is that the world is overwhelmingly absorbing the subtle negative image we have presented of parenting. To create a culture that values life, we must reaffirm the blessing that it is to steward little lives.

Does this mean we present parenting as easy and ourselves and children as flawless? Of course not. Authenticity will always have its place. What I *am* advocating is that we do not give an inordinate amount of air time to the difficulties of parenting even if those are the parts that get the most laughs or attention. Neither should we assume others understand the inherent joy that comes with the job. Someone who has never heard a toddler squeak out, "I love you so much, Mommy," will have difficulty understanding the life-altering power of such a small phrase. It is in those seemingly insignificant moments that a heart swells beyond what was thought possible and the resolve to make the world a better place for that little life is renewed. The world must see that we view parenting as a gift from God and that "every baby is a blessing," just as my father always said.

To take it one step further, our children need to see that too. Do we treat our children as blessings and acknowledge the honor it was to literally bear their image into the world? Do we speak to them in ways that reaffirm their worth to us? Are we respectful and genuine in our interactions with them? Are we reflecting the unconditional love of the Father, or do we withhold our affection when our kids don't meet our expectations? If we want the children in our homes and churches to value life, we must demonstrate to them through our words and actions that we recognize that they are gifts from God to us and that we are grateful to be entrusted with their lives.

All of my five children are beautiful image bearers. When they were young, they used to get magazines that often had a fun "Guess what this image is" activity on the back cover. There would be a series of pictures, all close-ups of a larger object: the fuzz of a tennis ball, the dimples of a dyed Easter egg, the fractals of a leaf. Some were easier than others, but they all proved this truth: It can be hard to define the reality of something when you are too close to it. Taking a step back can lend a whole new perspective to a situation. Beauty and chaos can look totally different depending on your view.

So it goes with a woman facing an unexpected pregnancy. In the moment, all one can see is the uncertainty, fear, self-doubt, and judgment. Society creates an image of a ruined future caused by a blob of tissue. But the zoe life says there is abundantly more. There is hope and beauty just on the other side of the chaos. My prayer is that people can take a moment to step back and look at the big picture. That "blob of tissue"? It is a unique human, full of possibilities just waiting to be realized. And the mother? Her future has the potential to be even more beautiful because of it. I know mine was.

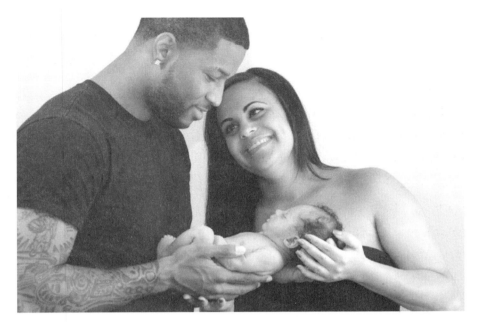

Amanda, Jeff & Hartlee

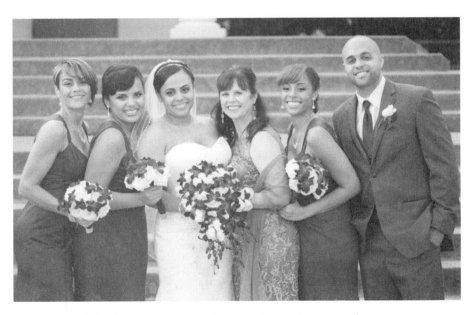

Laura & her 5 children: Arica, Mary, Amanda, Laura, Jazzi, Geoffrey
Photography by Mindy

CHAPTER 7

Abortion: When Death Becomes Vogue

Single parenting wasn't part of the pretty picture I had painted for myself. Even after I had Arica, I still had hopes that I would get married someday and live happily ever after. The marriage happened, but not the happily-ever-after part. When my marriages failed, I found myself alone, struggling to raise my five children. For years I provided day care so that I could stay home with them. When my last two entered school, I began a school photography business, so I wasn't able to be home as much as I would have liked, and my kids were at times unsupervised.

The summer before her freshman year in high school, my fourth child, Jazzi, and my youngest, Mary, were home alone one afternoon. When Jazzi's secret boyfriend showed up, he sent Mary and his cousin to play at the neighborhood park. Though he had shown signs of physical aggression in their eight months of dating, he had never forced her sexually… until then. She wished she had never opened the door. That afternoon, alone in her own house, Jazzi was raped. Her protests fell on deaf ears as tears streamed across her face. She became immobile and mute with fear.

Terrified—both of her boyfriend and of what people would say when they found out she was, as she felt, "damaged goods"—she kept the rape to herself, only telling her best friend. The sheer heartbreak I feel thinking about my baby going through that experience without me knowing and able to support her is sometimes debilitating. Shame is tricky like that. It sneaks in to silence and compound pain, when what is really needed is honesty and openness. Christine Caine puts it beautifully when she discusses the shame she felt as a result of her sexual abuse:

> *Why is it that the one sinned against feels that shame?*
> *Because sin, when unleashed, is so insidious, is such a*
> *violation of how we were created to live, that it often leaves*
> *the perpetrator and the victim, and even the witness, feeling*
> *stained.*[40]

A month after the assault, Jazzi missed her first period. Though her menstrual cycles were usually regular, she decided she was simply having an off month, not allowing herself to think about the alternative. When she missed her period for the second month in a row, however, she could no longer ignore the looming question in the back of her mind.

Am I pregnant? The thought overwhelmed her. She was fourteen—*fourteen*—and all signs were pointing to the reality that she might be pregnant with her rapist's baby. How was she supposed to process that?

She struggled under the weight of the implications. Up until that moment, Jazzi had been staunchly pro-life. She confidently discussed the topic of sanctity of life at all costs, and she certainly would not have said there were circumstances in which a woman was justified getting an abortion. But was she even a *woman?* She felt so much more like a girl—a lost girl, facing decisions way beyond her years. Two years before, she had zealously signed a pledge committing to save sex for marriage, to give it as a gift to her husband. When she was raped, that gift—that choice—had been ripped away from her, and she wondered if her future had been taken from her as well. Pregnant from rape at fourteen: not exactly the bright destiny she had imagined for herself. Faced with this stark reality, her arguments against abortion due to rape began to waiver. Now, it seemed, all bets were off.

Regardless of where each of us falls on the reproductive rights spectrum, we can all agree that situations in which women find themselves considering abortion are most often far from simple. The emotions that come into play with any unplanned pregnancy are complex and the negative physical or financial implications overwhelming. No matter the circumstance, it is never a choice made in a vacuum.

I would be doing a great disservice to those facing unplanned pregnancy, as well as the pro-life cause, by minimizing the seriousness of this decision or by dismissing the valid internal conflicts that arise in this situation.

Abortion touches us all. Even if we haven't personally had one performed, we swim in the ripples of its effects. According to the Center for Disease Control (CDC), annually, out of every one thousand live births, two hundred were ended in abortion.[41] When looking at the number of women, ages fifteen to forty-five, who have had at least one abortion, estimates range anywhere from one in five to one in three. With these numbers, it is evident that whether spoken or unspoken, each of us know women who have had an abortion. These numbers are consistent within the church. While it may be convenient to pretend that this is an issue outside of the church walls, it is only that—pretense.[42]

Regardless of where each of us falls on the reproductive rights spectrum, we can all agree that situations in which women find themselves considering abortion are most often far from simple. The emotions that come into play with any unplanned pregnancy are complex and the negative physical or financial implications overwhelming. No matter the circumstance, it is never a choice made in a vacuum.

I'm sure that right about now, some readers may be feeling pretty uncomfortable. Abortion is one of the most divisive and emotionally charged subjects today, and our culture at large is still trying to determine where exactly we stand on this issue. The topic of abortion has become so embroiled with politics, and politics has become such a flashpoint in the church, that we tend to avoid the discussion altogether out of fear of being associated with one political group over another or fear of its implications in our relationships and congregations. Still, as scary as approaching this can be, it's time to step outside our comfort zone and take a good hard look at the elephant in the room. I do not see how I can effectively talk about choosing a zoe life without focusing on this polarizing topic more fully.

While it will come as no surprise, my bottom line about abortion is that as a society we can do better. My views on this topic include, yet also go beyond, laws. They certainly do *not* include judging or shaming women who have had one. For me, it's about a better way—a zoe way. I have seen the effect abortions have on women's bodies and minds firsthand, and my ultimate goal here is to help women make choices that will spare them those negative and painful repercussions, as well as help women who have gone down this road to heal from guilt or shame. In order to do this, it is important that I dedicate this space to showing the ways in which abortion is a barrier to the zoe life.

Those who are parents will understand the weight of sorrow I feel when I share my daughter's rape story. We all want to protect our children, and my heart breaks when I think about situations in which

I was unable to do so. I know my parents would have done anything to protect me from my childhood molestation, had they known, or sought help for me afterward, like I did with Jazzi after she revealed her rape to a mandated reporter and I was then able to help her meet weekly with a Christian sexual trauma counselor for seven months. I wish I could go back to each time one of my children has suffered and take that pain from them, but I can't. What I can do is help heal the pain that already exists and prevent as much future pain as possible.

Current western culture promotes the idea that very little pain is associated with abortion, whether emotional or physical. I recently saw where a woman, a counselor at an abortion clinic herself, proudly filmed her abortion and then posted it on YouTube. Her reasoning for doing so was to show the world that abortion is a positive experience; it isn't scary or a big deal, and women shouldn't feel guilted by society or the pro-life movement.[43] She admits that she wasn't using any form of protection when she got pregnant, and thus the abortion was birth control. Despite this, she feels no guilt, is happy to report that the guy "wasn't involved" in the decision, and wants all women to know that her abortion experience was "special" and "as birth-like as it could be."

The sheer irony of some of her statements aside, especially the termination of a pregnancy being equated with bringing life into the world, this is a good example of culture normalizing abortion and hiding its true impact.Like the wolf in sheep's clothing, they dress death up in the language of life. I recently saw an advertisement for "abortion doula" training. Many women have expressed that they did not receive care or compassion at abortion clinics, even stating that they felt they were treated little better than cattle. The abortion industry is trying to address this accusation by creating a new position to fill this clear void—an acknowledgement that they have not been providing the care they have claimed. But an abortion doula is a poor counterfeit of the life-giving vocation of a birth doula. To compare the two is insulting at best.

Another example of cultural normalization comes from a source directly marketed to teens—a move I find telling of the abortion industry's intentions. In a *Teen Vogue* article titled "What to Get a Friend Post-Abortion," teens are told that deciding to have an abortion "is more than a little terrifying," but need not be scary.[44] "The worst part of all this," the article continues, "isn't the procedure itself (which by the way is completely safe as long as you have access to a good clinic). The worst part is how you're treated afterwards."

The sheer irony of some of her statements aside, especially the termination of a pregnancy being equated with bringing life into the world, this is a good example of culture normalizing abortion and hiding its true impact.

While the introduction itself doesn't blatantly state that abortion is "no big deal," the flippant language and suggestions certainly imply it. Teens are encouraged to commiserate with their friends on a level supposedly equal to the gravity of their situation. Watch a funny movie, give her gifts, such as a "girl power" cap, an "angry uterus" heating pad, a lapel pin with a uterus giving the middle finger (so people will know she doesn't regret her choice and—bonus!— proceeds go to abortion clinics). A needlepoint proclaiming "We Won't Go Back," coloring books, candy, or some special underwear ("technically they are made for your period, but that is no reason not to rock 'em for your post-abortion woes because there will be blood") are also suggested. If those don't do the trick, your friend could become an escort for other teens at abortion clinics, because "there is no better way to understand your own process than by helping someone else through it."

I agree with that last point—helping people go through a grief you have experienced yourself is indeed helpful and healing. What I disagree with is the inherent contradictions of the article, as well as the premise behind them that abortion is no big deal—like having wisdom teeth removed. Teens are told the only scary part is the treatment after the abortion, yet the heating pad is prescribed with this description of post-procedure symptoms: "It's like 2 throbbing hot balls of lead are trying to escape your body, all while your stomach contracts over and over again." That sounds pretty scary. And if the atmosphere outside an abortion clinic is as terrifying as the abortion movement claims, advocating teens to repeatedly put themselves in that situation seems irresponsible at best. Further, choosing an abortion is equated with having "Girl Power," but what then should a girl feel who carries her pregnancy to term? Is she not powerful? Some would say it is the right to a *choice* that makes her powerful, but I have yet to see a similar article lauding a teen who *chooses* to give her baby up for adoption.

A woman is perfectly within her legal right to terminate her pregnancy. But is there room in legality for mercy and compassion? And just because something is legal, does that make it right? Is there not a better way? Is the power of having a choice enough to cover the act itself? How has death become vogue, when we are fashioned for life?

The article by *Teen Vogue* is not the enemy; there are many more like it elsewhere. Still, it reveals the blatant attempt by our mainstream culture to trivialize abortion and its effects on women (and men!). It is not a minor procedure made better by a heating pad. An outspoken element of the pro-choice movement will tout the inconsequential nature of an abortion, but there are many women in that same movement who would disagree. While they still advocate for the right to an abortion, they acknowledge that the act carries with it great meaning and consequence, and to treat it in such a flippant way is to negate the deep emotions women have surrounding this choice. Far and wide, the women I speak to do not seem proud— or glad—of this decision, and it isn't because they are ashamed to admit it. It is because they have genuine sadness.

These aren't testimonies only from people in the pro-life movement. Women with no obvious agenda have spoken out about their detrimental abortion experiences, as is the case of another young woman who posted her abortion story on YouTube. While the woman who filmed her abortion was clearly trying to make a statement for her industry, this second video was much more raw and honest. This young woman speaks about how sure she is she made the right decision, but as she recounts her experience, grief is written on every line of her face and sounds in every note in her voice. It's as though she is trying to convince herself. She is so obviously hurting, I want to reach through the screen and hug her, but I can't. What I *can* do is try to keep another girl from being in that same place.

Abortion laws have made the ability to do this more difficult, especially when it comes to protecting young girls. In over twenty-five states, including my state of California, minors are not required to have parental consent to have an abortion, and in many of them, parents are not even notified, regardless of age. In those states that do require parental permission, abortion advocates are quick to point out that a judge can waive that requirement.[45] In my work at the pregnancy resource center, in a single month I encountered three twelve-year-old girls who were pregnant.

Twelve.

Years.

Old.

People may chuckle or dismiss Jazzi for making a vow of chastity at the age of twelve, but girls younger than that are getting pregnant. Clearly vows like this are important. Abortion advocates are quick to point out a woman's right to choose, but is a twelve-year-old a *woman?* Is she equipped to deal with such a traumatic thing as a pregnancy, let alone an abortion, on her own? Laws removing parental involvement at any age suggest that, yes, indeed a twelve-year-old is equipped to make such choices. Our society doesn't allow someone under the age of eighteen to buy cough syrup, but we think it is okay for pre-teens to decide and abort by themselves. By law in

Illinois, children under the age of fourteen are not allowed to stay home alone, yet they are not required to have parental consent for an abortion as a minor. My heart breaks for these children because that is what they are—children—and they need their parents.

To make matters worse, in many cases these pregnancies are a result of abuse. As a volunteer, I am a mandated reporter. I want to get these girls out of abusive situations, and I try my hardest to do so. Unfortunately, though abortion clinics are technically mandated reporters, they also have a "Don't Ask, Don't Tell" policy. Evidence suggests that they neglect reporting because, to put it crudely, it would cut too far into their bottom line.[46] On top of the trauma of pregnancy and abortion, these children are sent back into the same environments that got them there to begin with.

Not only is the pain associated with abortion downplayed and the fine print of abortion laws obscured, the prevalence and economic impact is as well. Camouflaged under the generic term of "women's reproductive health," the nation's leading abortion provider maintains that only 3 percent of its services are accounted for by abortion.[47] That figure would make it appear that very little of what the organization does is actually abortion. That percentage is technically true, but only because every service is considered separate and given equal weight. A urine test is the same as an abortion. Hypothetically speaking, if a woman comes in for an abortion, she is likely to have a pregnancy test, one or more medications, a blood test, possible anesthesia, and perhaps a prescription for birth control. Her appointment would involve these seven services, only one of which is an abortion. However, it's abortion, not the pain pill, that will stick in her mind. It is easy to see how skewed the 3 percent claim is.[48]

Further, the abortion industry is bound by the Hyde Amendment, which prohibits federal funding to directly pay for abortions. Instead, the leading abortion provider uses the 43 percent of its income provided by government funding to cover non-abortion costs. This frees up clinic fees and private donations to fund abortions and generate their profit.[49] As much as I want to spend all my income on baby clothes, the necessity of running a small business, paying my mortgage, insurance, and grocery bills limits how much I can spend on the latest fashions. However, if a wealthy benefactor came along and agreed to pay for all my living necessities, just *think* of how much income I would have at my disposal for clothes!

With the cost of a medication-induced abortion at $800 and a procedural abortion at $1,500, if one organization's report of 323,999 abortions in one year is accurate, more than $485 million comes in from abortions alone.[50] No wonder the abortion industry is so aggressively marketing and normalizing it. With few overhead expenses, thanks to the Federal Government, abortion is a cash cow.

With such a lucrative business at its fingertips, the "women's reproductive health movement" has great incentive to minimize any of abortion's ill effects. The continued assertions on all levels that abortion is completely safe, with little to no side-effects, belies its true toll on the human body. Emotional and physical trauma aside (which I will deal with in the next chapter), abortion carries with it a much higher physical risk than the industry would like to acknowledge. To begin with, abortion-related deaths are often underreported because actual cause of death is usually coded by the hospital. If the patient died of hemorrhaging from an abortion, then hemorrhaging, not the abortion, would be recorded. According to a 2004 study:

In the American Journal of Obstetrics and Gynecology, 2004; the mortality rate associated with abortion is 2.95 times higher than that associated with pregnancies carried to term. Non-pregnant women had 57.0 deaths per 100,000, compared to 28.2 for women who carried to term, 51.9 for women who miscarried, and 83.1 for women who had abortions. A 46% higher death rate than non-pregnant women. The study also revealed a seven-fold increased rate of deaths from suicide among aborting women. The study included the entire population of women 15 to 49 years of age in Finland between 1987 and 2000. This same study was also published in the European Journal of Public Health 15(5):459-63 (2005). Stating that compared to women who have not been pregnant in the prior year, deaths from suicide, accidents and homicide are 428% higher in the year following an abortion. The publication also noted that the majority of extra deaths among post-abortive women were due to suicide. The suicide rate among post-abortive women was six times higher than that of women who had given birth in the prior year and double that of women who had miscarriages. The risk of death was lowest among women who gave birth within the prior year.[51]

Furthermore, the abortion industry claims that previous

abortions and D&C's have no effect on future fertility. However, one doctor I spoke to who specializes in reproductive endocrinology and infertility says that when dealing with an ectopic pregnancy or situation in which dead fetal tissue must be removed from the mother, D&C's are usually the last resort because they pose such a great risk of uterine scarring and therefore further infertility issues.[52]

There is much more that could be said regarding specific arguments against abortion and the physical danger it poses, but I don't want to get so bogged down in the details and arguments that the big picture gets lost. There are plenty of resources that go into more depth on these topics, and I encourage those interested to see the resources listed at the end of this book and to do further research.

Dr. Kathi Aultman knows all too well the pull of the abortion industry and its hidden physical and emotional effect on women. A doctor with specialized training in late-term abortions, Dr. Aultman spent years performing abortions out of a conviction that abortion on demand was a woman's right and an unwanted child was better off not being born. In her testimony to Congress, Dr. Aultman states that a combination of things began to change her mind. First, during her neonatal care rotations she found herself trying to save babies who were the same gestation age of those she was aborting. Further, her interactions with women who unapologetically used abortion as birth control and even seemed hostile toward the fetus growing within them were in stark contrast to the women who mourned terminating their pregnancies. Finally, the juxtaposition of successful and happy women who chose to keep their babies with the continued mental and physical trauma of those who had chosen abortion painted a picture of the often severe consequences of abortion. Whether or not a child was wanted was no longer a justification for her killing it. While she believes that a woman needs "as much choice as possible in determining her future and what she does with her body," society "must also recognize the truth that there are at least 2 people involved in a pregnancy and that at some point the rights of the weaker one deserve some consideration."[53]

This consideration of the "weaker one" can be especially difficult in the case of maternal health. Delivered on the same day as the infamous *Roe v. Wade,* the case of *Doe v. Bolton* is often overlooked. While *Roe* legalized abortion, *Doe* struck down the gestation limitations regarding what stage of pregnancy abortions could be performed in, as long as it was deemed "necessary to the health of the mother." The ruling allowed for abortions to be performed after the age of viability—where a child could live outside of the womb—even up until birth if the mother's health was affected. The provisions were further broadened by the definition of "health of the mother":

> *…the medical judgment may be exercised in the light of all factors—physical, emotional, psychological, familial, and the woman's age—relevant to the well-being of the patient. All these factors may relate to health.*[54]

The vagueness of the definition essentially removed any true barrier to late-term abortion, because almost anything could be related back to the mother's health. As such, there are many women who have ended pregnancies after the age of viability simply because they were unwanted. But what about the women who ended their pregnancies with heartache, knowing what it is to love or long for a child? What about the women who were told they had to make a choice between giving birth to the child in their womb or being a parent to the ones they already had? These are seemingly impossible situations, and no pat answer does them justice.

When I was pregnant with my second child, Geoffrey, I had complications that required two surgeries, and in order to carry, I was bedridden during the entire pregnancy. The pregnancy was a serious strain on my body and my marriage. It was a difficult time for all of us, and I am thankful for a medical staff who worked diligently to help me find a way to keep my pregnancy.

I was not told I had to choose, but I know there are many women who have been given that devastating news. My friend Serena is one of them. At twenty weeks pregnant, doctors told her that her baby had Alpha Thalassemia Major, a severe genetic blood disorder. Her baby was unable to make the required amount of healthy blood, and was therefore trying to use Serena's. Tests showed that the effects of this had already begun to take a toll on her baby and that she was dying in the womb. Matters were further complicated by Serena's own genetic blood issues and she was beginning to show signs of preeclampsia. Doctors told Serena and her husband that continuing the pregnancy would severely endanger Serena's life, and her baby's chances of survival were low even if she did. They urged her to do a D&C. The choice was excruciating, and she couldn't bear the thought of having her baby ripped apart inside of her. But Serena had another child to think about, and in the end she requested that the doctors induce labor so that she could give a live birth to her baby and give her a chance at survival. Labor was intense and all the more excruciating knowing the likely outcome for her child. Their daughter Alexa was born, and the family had one beautiful hour with her, bonding and taking photos, before she took her last breath. Serena and her husband are grateful that they pushed beyond the options given to them and gave their daughter what small chance she might have had at life.[55]

Choosing a course of action in such a dark time is deeply personal and between a mother and father, but I would urge those facing such a daunting decision to push medical staff to *really* consider all the options. Often the medical community will do what seems to be the proven path of least resistance. Dedication to the best care for their patients, as well as the ever-present threat of malpractice lawsuits, influence this course of action that isn't always the best for the patient either. However, when another life is at stake, the usual playbook doesn't always cut it. Doctors need to be driven to look for solutions that don't involve ending the pregnancy—they are often out there! I was recently told of a couple in Colorado who had two children and were expecting their third. The mother was having serious complications and was told that she needed to terminate her pregnancy. They were devastated. After seeking counsel, they approached the medical staff and asked what they would do for the pregnancy if abortion wasn't an option. The medical staff went back to the drawing board and came up with a solution that allowed the mother to safely carry her pregnancy to term and deliver a healthy child. The mother was on bedrest for several months, and their church community surrounded them and provided the additional support they needed. In the end, the caring and compassionate medical staff was grateful because they had been forced to find a life-saving solution where they had, in the past, turned to abortion.[56]

These are weighty choices, and I don't want to stand in judgment or heap pain where there already is so much. But I will say that when parents live a zoe life and do all they can to provide that to their child, there can be peace, and there can be miracles.

It was with this same hope that my daughter Jazzi made the decision to keep her baby. She decided to step outside of what happened to her and focus on what she was creating. She knew God loved her and was going to partner with her. Yes, half of her baby's DNA would be her rapist's, but her child would be wholly God's, and He would help her sustain her pregnancy. God cared about what happened to her, and her future was not destroyed. She was not damaged goods. She knew that she couldn't judge all men by her rapist, and someday she would meet a man who loved her and wanted to be a father to her child.

She felt firm in her decision, yet still scared. Then one day at school, three months after her rape, she got her period. She wasn't pregnant after all. The trauma of the event had caused her body to go haywire for a few months. Jazzi chose zoe, and even though she turned out not to be pregnant, that choice stuck, and it has influenced her life and the lives of others. She now helps girls and women recover from sexual trauma by giving her testimony, speaking in high schools about dating violence, and preaching, teaching, and sharing at churches and conferences. I'm so grateful for her boldness and her sweet heart to want to see people protected and healed. Jazzi has overcome by the blood of the Lamb and the power of her testimony.

"Ah," some might say, "your anecdote is flawed. She wasn't pregnant. It doesn't count." Let me tell you another. Remember my friend Serena, who chose to give birth to her dying daughter? When she was seven years old, her uncle, a priest in training, began raping her. She told her parents about it, but they said she was lying—it wasn't possible.

"Silence, Serena. Be quiet."

"You are a worthless disappointment."

"Lies."

"You want to ruin our family."

"Hush."

So for four years she was raped, until her uncle died when she was eleven. I can't imagine the amount of emotional trauma forced on her at such a young age and the isolation she must have felt at her parents' betrayal.

When she was fourteen, she was walking with her boyfriend around the deserted grounds of her high school after they had both stayed late for various school functions. She was a freshman, he a senior. She was wearing her favorite pleated skirt and blouse, knee high socks, and suspenders. When they came to a women's restroom, her boyfriend said he needed to use it.

"You can't go in there," Serena said, "that's the women's restroom."

"Oh, it's fine. You should come in with me," he laughed.

"No. I don't feel comfortable with that."

"Come in with me."

"No."

At that point, he grabbed her and forced her into the bathroom and pushed her into the stall. She fought, but he was so much stronger. She pleaded. She begged. She yelled.

"Silence, Serena. Be quiet. You are worthless."

After he raped her, he left her there, clothes in tatters.

She went home and told her mother.

"Well, that's what you get for wearing what you're wearing."

Alone—utterly alone—she stumbled through the next few months. She closed herself off from everyone. She removed all traces of vulnerability. Five months after the assault, a terrible pain in her side made her go to the doctor.

"Did you know you were pregnant?" the doctor asked.

"What? How can that be? I haven't missed my period."

"Sometimes that happens." The doctor encouraged her to have a D&C. After all, she was too young to have a baby. Serena went home and told her parents. And no surprise, they were anything but supportive. They, too, told her to have an abortion even though it was against their strict religious views.

"You are a worthless disappointment, Serena."

"This baby will ruin your life."

But she couldn't abort him. She had felt him *move*. That thing inside of her was a living, moving being. None of this was his fault. He was a part of her.

She kept her baby, and for the next few months endured the scorn so often given to pregnant teens. She found it especially difficult in her church, where the message of choosing life had been so strong, yet when it was obvious she was doing just that, she was met with disdain. She does note, thankfully, that there were some who praised her for her choice, but those people were few and far between.

Giving birth to her son was one of the best decisions she has ever made. She had to continually fight for him to have a childhood different from her own. Her parents did not change. While they begrudgingly helped her raise him when she was young, they continued to heap shame on her and her son. One day, in a fit of frustration, her father yelled at her son, "You weren't wanted! You were born out of rape! We told your mother to abort you. You aren't even supposed to be here!"

Despite the abuse and anguish, Serena and her son made a life together. She says that having her son and persevering on his behalf is why she is even alive today. Without him, she fears the pain would have been too great and she would have given up.

Serena eventually met and married a man who loved her *and* her son and raised him as his own. Together they weathered the death of their daughter and have the security of all being reunited one day. Through it all, her son was at her side, giving her hope and courage.

"He is my blessing. My blessing I didn't know I needed," she says of her son. There was power in her choice of choosing zoe and continuing her pregnancy in the midst of seemingly hopeless circumstances.

Speak life, Serena.

You are strong and brave and make this world a better place.

You are wonderfully made and have created something beautiful.

CHAPTER 8

Healing from Abortion

Somewhere on the other side of her wall, Ethel could hear a baby crying. She was sure of it. Day and night, he wouldn't stop. How could that be? There were no babies who lived in her nursing home. Still, he cried. Why was no one helping him? Was he crying for her? He was! He was crying for her! She needed to help him! She would save him. She began to beat on the wall, but it did not budge. At eighty years of age her body no longer held the strength it once did. She began to dig. She clawed at the drywall. She did not stop when the first cut appeared, nor the second. By the time the nursing staff came to intervene, she had dug into the drywall, exposing her fingers almost to the bone.

Ethel would not be consoled. The baby was counting on her, and she was failing him. After several weeks and multiple attempts to calm her and convince her there was no baby in need of her help, the nursing and psychiatric staff finally called a meeting with her family.

Her children had no idea what could be causing the delusions and outbursts, and her husband said he could not help. Ethel continued to fight to get to the child on the other side of the wall and was distraught at her inability to do so.

A few days after the initial meeting with the family, Ethel's husband called to speak with her geriatric psychiatrist. He needed someone to talk to. As the story spilled out of him, the psychiatrist began to see a reason for his wife's delusions.

Decades earlier, during the Depression, he and Ethel were struggling to survive and feed their four children. When they discovered Ethel was pregnant with their fifth child, he insisted she have an abortion. How would they all survive if they had another mouth to feed? He felt there was no choice. *Did the psychiatrist see there had been no choice?*

Armed with this knowledge, the psychiatrist began a course of treatment that proved effective. Ethel was given a life-sized baby doll and told it was her baby and that she was to care for it. Her tears ceased. She no longer heard a phantom baby cry or harmed herself. The psychiatrist believes this was because Ethel was given a chance to care for the baby she had been denied so many years earlier. The grief of that decision had weighed on her for decades—from the 1930s until now, the 1980s—toying with her self-worth and eventually her mental faculties.[57]

This was the story I was told by that same geriatric psychiatrist when I asked her if she thought Post Abortion Stress Syndrome was real. Post Abortion Stress Syndrome (PAS), related to Post Traumatic Stress Disorder (PTSD), is the term that describes the psychological aftereffects of abortion.[58] Many in the pro-choice movement deny its existence, claiming it is a term created by the pro-life movement to strike fear into the hearts of women. The reality is that PAS is a very real condition. It was real for Ethel, and it is real for thousands of others. Even medical publications, with clear bias toward the pro-choice movement, declare that post-abortion trauma does exist.[59]

The symptoms of PAS are similar to those of PTSD: depression, anxiety, shame, feelings of isolation or self-harm, compulsive or addictive behaviors, nightmares, anger, sexual dysfunction, trouble bonding in relationships, and eating disorders, to name a few. This is a valid, proven condition, and it can be devastating.

It's hard to argue with the statistics. The organization Silent No More has done an excellent job compiling some of the most compelling ones, and following are just a few. According to a 2006 New Zealand study, of the women in the study group, 42% who had an abortion experienced major depression at a 35% higher rate than the women who carried their pregnancies to term. A study published in the *Canadian Medical Association Journal* stated that the rate of psychiatric hospitalization was 2.6 times higher in every time period examined for women who had abortions compared with women who continued with their pregnancies. In California, a study of 173,000 women found that those who had abortions were 63% more likely to receive mental care within 90 days of the event compared to women who gave birth, and that rates of continued mental health treatment were significantly higher for the women who had aborted. In another sample of 10,847 women who had no history of anxiety prior to their unplanned pregnancy, those who aborted were 30% more likely to report symptoms consistent with generalized anxiety disorder. Finally (I know! So many numbers!), according to a 2006 article in the *Journal of Youth and Adolescence*, adolescent girls who abort unplanned pregnancies versus those who keep them are five times more likely to pursue help for emotional and psychological problems, three times more likely to report sleep issues, and nine times more likely to be advised of marijuana use.[60] Many of these findings were corroborated by a subsequent study published in 2011 by the *British Journal of Psychiatry*.[61]

Georgette Forney, President of Silent No More, herself had an abortion at the age of sixteen. As one can imagine, she has received a lot of negative attention from abortion advocates for her work in the pro-life arena. After one particularly scathing article was published, attacking her own psychological well-being and discounting the notion that there is pain associated with abortion, Georgette's daughter beautifully summed up the issue when she said, "Mom, their research says women aren't hurting, but you work seven days a week to help the women they say don't exist."[62]

There is a certain amount of preaching to the choir here, I realize that. But my intent for including these statistics (of which there are many, many more) is two-fold. First, I believe it is important that women who are experiencing these symptoms realize they are not alone. Second, the people on the fence about abortion need to acknowledge that there are serious consequences—not just to the child, but the mother as well. If people are truly pro-women's health, promoting a practice that has demonstrated dire consequences to both the physical and psychological health of women makes absolutely no sense. And ignoring the actual physical and emotional effects in an effort to promote an agenda is irresponsible at best.

While I have told the story of my fourth child, Jazzi, who was faced with making a decision of life and death, my first baby, Arica, whom I chose to keep at fifteen years of age, made a decision unknown to me at the time that led her into twenty years of stuffed emotional pain.

My first husband adopted Arica, and she has always considered him her father. But when she was ten, our marriage dissolved, and Arica was left reeling. The changed nature of our family unit, combined with the latent feelings of abandonment from her biological father, led Arica to notice attention of older males. Saddened at her dad's decreased presence in her life and unwilling to have me aware of surrounding influences, she hid these advances and interests and was unprepared to deal with the manipulation and sexual pressures that came with them. I had not built that important relationship of openness and communication with Arica, and I always naively assumed the best. She spent her time with friends— friends who came from families with convictions much different than mine.

At the age of seventeen, she discovered she was pregnant. She was scared. She wanted everything to stay the way it had been— continuing her social life, her athletics, and her career path. As she says,

I respected my mom so much for giving birth to me, even though she was a teen. But I saw how hard she had to

work, and the sacrifices she had to make, and I just didn't think I was strong enough. I wasn't good enough for my own biological father to get it together. I wasn't good enough for my parents to find a way to save their marriage. I wasn't good enough to be a mom.[63]

So she turned to a friend for advice. This friend willingly walked Arica through the all too familiar process. At the time, Arica was too consumed with her own turmoil to make the connection between her friend's brokenness due to abortion and her friend's subsequent substance abuse.

Arica took the city bus to her first appointment at the local reproductive women's health clinic. She took the pregnancy test and then sat in the waiting room. She felt gross and detached, partly from the fear of being found out and partly from the cold atmosphere in the room. When she was called back, there was very little conversation. Everything was businesslike. They asked if the pregnancy was wanted or unwanted. When Arica told them it was unexpected, they presumed to immediately book her for the next available abortion, emphasizing the importance of getting it done before she was further along and the fees increased.

The day of her abortion, her friend drove her to the clinic. The doctor was cold and aloof, and Arica wondered if she was even qualified to perform the procedure. Afterwards, they gave her an icepack and sent her on her way. Afraid of people finding out, she went back to school and completed her softball practice. Standing there in the field, bleeding, in physical and emotional pain, she remembers hearing the other girls laugh and carry on as usual. It was jarring.

For the two weeks leading up to the abortion, Arica grieved her decision. But once it was done, she stuffed the pain. How could she allow herself to grieve a decision she willingly made even when she knew it was wrong? She would not give herself the permission. Instead, she determined to carefully control her life for the best. In her mind, she had denied her baby a chance at life because of her career aspirations, so she better have the best career possible. Subconsciously, she could never be good enough. Her self-judgment and shame left her feeling "less than" in every area of her life and over the years began poisoning her marriage and making it hard for her to connect with her young children. Ironically, in an effort to avoid the dysfunction and pain of the teen parent life, she introduced deep pain and dysfunction into other areas of her life. She didn't even feel like she was good enough to truly commune with God. She struggled with seeing God as a father whom she could trust to protect her, because no one in her life had consistently done so, and yet neither had she for her child. The reality of the hurtful, dysfunctional cycle that affected her decision to abort kept her distant from both God and others. She did not acknowledge that abortion does not remove all the consequences of teen pregnancy.

After over a decade of trying to force her way to success, despondent in her career, with a marriage on the brink of disaster, she sought help. With the original intent of working through issues in her marriage, she joined a support group. What she discovered in that group, however, was how tied the problems in her life were to her childhood perceptions, her abortion experience, and the resulting guilt, shame, and need to perform. She had been frantically managing her life on all levels in an attempt to make up for aborting her baby.

The day of her abortion, her friend drove her to the clinic. The doctor was cold and aloof, and Arica wondered if she was even qualified to perform the procedure. Afterwards, they gave her an icepack and sent her on her way. Afraid of people finding out, she went back to school and completed her softball practice. Standing there in the field, bleeding, in physical and emotional pain, she remembers hearing the other girls laugh and carry on as usual. It was jarring.

As she began to take steps to heal, Arica had a vision of her heart in a beautiful, sparkling glass box with gold trim. The box was stunning, but her heart was entangled in chains. The question she kept hearing was: *Do you trust the Lord with your heart?* She desperately wanted to, and the Lord met her vulnerability. He lifted her heart, and the chains fell away. The Holy Spirit later revealed an image of Jesus, larger than life, leaning down and gently carrying her over the shattered remains of a bridge that had been her life and setting her solidly on the other side. She knew He forgave her of every incident from her past. She could sense the reality that Jesus loves women who have had abortions and those who have fallen into mental and emotional traps, that He is waiting to forgive them and bring healing. She leaned into this truth.

It was much harder, though, to forgive herself. She felt she had knowingly inflicted this damage, so why should she deserve reconciliation? When someone has been wronged, they instinctively seek retribution. But she couldn't conceive how to make right something so wrong. How do you seek retribution against yourself? She was not alone in this struggle. Many women report having felt guilt over their abortions and therefore punishing themselves. Whether the refusal to have more children, neglect of their physical bodies, self-limiting affection with subsequent children, or realizing the possible connection between their abortion and subsequent infertility issues, this self-punishment can heap pain upon pain. It is an act of self-retribution, a subliminal penance.

As she leaned into the truth of God's forgiveness, she began to realize a second truth: Who was she to deny the forgiveness that God lovingly offered? How could she have the audacity to view herself and her choices as bigger than Christ and the cross? Yes, He loved the child she had aborted, but He also loved her—she, too, was His creation. Denying herself His grace and mercy stood in the way of His plan for her life. Slowly, she stopped seeking retribution against herself and made a conscious effort to let herself off the hook.

At the advice of a counselor, she began seeking out the things that had given her joy when she was young and untainted by life's traumas. She rediscovered her passion for artistic creativity and gave herself grace not to be perfect in those endeavors. Reconnecting with those long-denied, God-given passions rekindled her joy.

Finally, after coming to terms with her own failings and God's forgiveness, she has worked through her grief to the point she is able to help guide others through theirs. Now, years after she began her healing, she continues to actively lead a Celebrate Recovery group and guide others on this journey. Helping other women and men through their pain has been a continued source of healing and rejuvenation for her. As she describes, "I feel like, in some ways, I had to make some of the worst mistakes in life to truly understand God's forgiveness and learn not to condemn others. I can't help but want to help others break through their pain and find real freedom."

For Arica, as for many women I've spoken to, one of the most difficult parts of being post-abortive is the knowledge that so few know this huge thing about your life and the feeling that they wouldn't understand even if they did. Arica felt alone in her pain. As her mother, this saddens me. Through her post-abortive recovery, however, she came to realize that God had seen her pain and had bottled up her tears; they had not been in vain, and she had never been alone.

Often women are scared to mourn. They are afraid that revisiting the memory will open a Pandora's box of negative feelings. They will scratch the surface—perhaps go to an informational meeting—but even if there is an option for in-depth counseling or group therapy, they won't take advantage of it. The thought of confronting the pain is too much. This can be especially true of women who were forced to have abortions or men who were given no say in the choice of what happened to their child. They can't face their grief, and it eats away at their soul.

Grief. The word itself hits me in the gut. Our world is full of it. The sin that began as disobedience in the Garden of Eden has followed us through the millennia, digging its claws in wherever it can, causing misery and pain. Academics have tried to loosely organize it into various stages, with labels such as: denial, rage, depression, and acceptance. Of course, not everyone agrees on how many stages there are, what to call them, or how to cycle through them, because *everyone grieves differently.*

No one can prescribe how another person should grieve. For some, grief can feel like an insurmountable obstacle, a Mt. Everest standing between them and a normal, happy life. For others, the stages seem to flow quickly and naturally. Whatever way grieving happens, it is important that it does, indeed, *happen.*

It is only through facing the pain that people can truly overcome it. Living in denial opens doors to addictions.

Efforts to distract cannot bring hoped-for relief and result in additional pain and stress. In order to avoid pain, people learn to deny it is even there, and that denial fuels the anxiety, depression, sleep disorders, phobias, and addictions that seem to plague our society today. Pain is the root of so much evil in the world—the opposite of what God intended for His creation. But there is hope. God can break that denial and bring healing, opening the door to zoe. The abundant life is waiting, and freedom from guilt and shame are within reach, but first the pain must be faced and truly grieved.

It is only through facing the pain that people can truly overcome it. Living in denial opens doors to addictions.

As a mother and grandmother, this is what I had to do in my own life when I learned of Arica's abortion. I felt as if a huge weight had been placed on my chest. Grief for a lost grandchild and knowing my daughter had to experience abortion alone crushed me emotionally and left me gasping for air.

But...

But God is ever the One who brings beauty out of the ashes. In my grieving process, I cried out to Him to help me fight the injustice. Two days after this prayer, I was asked to speak at an event for a state program whose funding is funneled through abortion clinics. God gave me a platform, literally, to share my story with pregnant teens, new parents, local dignitaries, and abortion clinic staff and advocates. Like my father before me, I encouraged others to choose life, an education, and Jesus. Using the Virgin Mary as an example, I emphasized that we never know the gift we are carrying.

I faced my pain, and God used it to fuel my passion and courage to save countless more women and their babies. What was meant for harm and destruction, God salvaged and used for beauty. Jesus has lifted my heavy burden, and I rejoice that I can observe my beautiful, healed daughter leading others to the zoe life and will one day meet my grandchild.

Just like me, Arica had to go on her own journey of healing. For women and men facing post-abortive grief, the ministry of Rachel's Vineyard has been an important one. Designed as a weekend retreat, those touched by the loss of abortion (parents, grandparents, siblings) are led through carefully orchestrated steps to help them address the grief associated with abortion and to begin healing. It is a wonderful retreat opportunity available throughout the United States and in several countries, and I highly recommend it. Arica experienced this healing firsthand when she attended with her husband, who wanted to better understand her pain.

My son-in-law was not the lone male at Rachel's Vineyard. Many men struggle with post-abortive pain and grieve their aborted children. While I acknowledge the importance of women having good healthcare and not being subjected to the medical whims of men, I do not believe abortion falls into this category. Resisting abortion is not about grabbing power; it's about human rights. Someone advocating for refugees isn't told they are trying to control someone else's life—their struggle is recognized as a humanitarian effort. The argument that resistance to abortion is really just about men wanting to control women's bodies is, in fact, a tired one. I would argue that power-seeking men actually have far more to gain from the prevalence of abortion than they do from its decline: fewer restrictions on their lives and sexual prowess, less child support and thus more financial freedom, etc.

The prevailing push toward women's physical autonomy has reduced men to mere sperm donors and limited their importance and, dare I say, *right* to be a part of choices made regarding their unborn children.

Men have been told that because it isn't their body carrying the pregnancy, they have no say in the decision. This is tragic. There are fathers out there—some whom I know—who have stepped up to raise their children as single parents or helped throughout the pregnancy and assisted in placing the child for adoption, who have stood by their women and made a family work. There are many more who wish they'd been given the chance.

There is a song that I think sums up beautifully the pain felt from abortion. The artist is not making any political statement on the right to choose—I'm not sure if he is pro-life or pro-choice—but he is honest and raw about his experience and equates it to "drowning slowly." He discusses taking his girlfriend to an abortion clinic while her parents are out of town, and the utter loneliness they both feel, even though they have "finally found someone." After he drops her at the abortion clinic, he kills time in the parking lot (because women are forced to endure this experience on their own), and then goes to sell the gifts he had already purchased for his baby. "Can't you see? It's not me you're dying for!" he plaintively tells his child. It's heartbreaking.[64]

What I am advocating is far from any sort of propaganda meant to assert male dominance over women. I am advocating simply that parents be allowed to protect their children, whether that parent be male or female. Contrary to current societal trends and pushes from the media, men are not the enemy. We need to stop demonizing them. I firmly believe treating men with respect and expecting responsibility will cause more men to stand up and take action on behalf of their families. Do I think men should be able to dominate women and control them? No. Do I think they need to be heard? Absolutely. Their expressions of grief are just as valid, as is their need to receive forgiveness and healing.[iii]

Men have been told that because it isn't their body carrying the pregnancy, they have no say in the decision. This is tragic. There are fathers out there—some whom I know— who have stepped up to raise their children as single parents or helped throughout the pregnancy and assisted in placing the child for adoption, who have stood by their women and made a family work. There are many more who wish they'd been given the chance.

Some would say that the grief or trauma associated with abortion is the result of guilt and shame heaped upon them by the religious community. Based on the many women with whom I have spoken and the countless others of whom I've read, I would argue that a tremendous amount of grief is inherent in the choice to have an abortion and this idea that shame comes only because of the religious community is just a convenient scapegoat. Human nature is such that we try to find anything and anyone to point the finger of blame at if it

---

iii   Resources for such healing are included in Appendices B and C at the back of this book.

means avoiding pointing it at ourselves. That said, I would also agree that there are those in the religious community who have handled this very badly. In some cases, the grief women feel from an abortion has been intensified by the reactions of others. For many, the shame of admitting to an abortion and the possible backlash in the religious community has led women to hide their pain, and therefore not get healing.

Georgette Forney recently told me of an encounter she had with a woman who had an abortion. They were at a pro-life rally, and the woman opened up to Georgette about the pain her abortion had caused. When Georgette suggested she stand with the men and women who were publicly stating they regretted their abortions, she was horrified. She didn't want anyone from her church community in attendance to know she had actually had an abortion. She was convinced they would see her differently and perhaps even ostracize her.[65] Sadly, this is the case for many in the church, so let me be clear: Women who have had abortions are just as loved by God and just as worthy of forgiveness as the rest of us, who have all sinned. Redemption covers us all.

So, what can the church do to change this? First, we need to acknowledge the true state of affairs. Statistics show that between one in three or one in five women have had an abortion, and with 70 percent of them self-identifying as Christians at the time of their abortion, it is likely that there are women, perhaps many, sitting in our congregations, week after week, suffering from pain and regret. Some may feel they have no lasting impact from the abortion, but others are grieving in silence, perhaps to the extent of addiction. The church cannot, in good conscience, ignore this epidemic any longer. While Pope Francis may have extended the 2016 year of mercy for those who have had abortions in the Catholic Church, I believe God's mercy is forever available and always a wise path to follow. Pastors who wish to educate themselves can review the resources listed within the appendices at the end of this book.

Once church leadership has acknowledged the prevalence of this pain and educated themselves, they are prepared to take further action. My church, Liberty, under the direction of Pastor Joan West, has done a phenomenal job with this and even developed steps to help other churches succeed. While the information below has been successful in my church, I know that solutions are not always one-size-fits-all. Churches should prayerfully consider options that will work best in their communities.

Step 1: Develop a team

Church leadership should begin by developing a team of both women and men who are passionate about helping others heal from abortion through serving as leaders for a ten-week healing process. Team members should attend post-abortive trainings and grief seminars and pray continually for new insights to reach those affected by abortion. The hope is that people will experience healing and in turn be trained to lead their own healing group.

Step 2: Develop effective outreach using existing ministries

Church ministries, such as recovery programs, counseling, and in-depth, team-led prayer sessions, may present opportunities for post-abortive healing and recovery for those who have participated in abortion. Educate ministry leaders to encourage people who are suffering to come forward for help with healing.

Step 3: Demonstrate compassionate church awareness

As scary as it may seem, church leadership needs to be bold in addressing the topic of abortion, and the need for post-abortive healing. Simply ignoring it will not make it go away; it will just fester. Because some women were coerced into abortion by the men in their lives, and so it is helpful to have a female pastor or a spiritually mature woman involved in presenting this topic.

When my pastors started their abortion-healing ministry, A Movement of Love, they spoke together as senior pastors to the entire congregation, educating us regarding the scientific and spiritual facts about life beginning at the moment of conception. They compassionately helped our congregation understand that abortion is not God's will and He will forgive and heal those who have had them or partnered with them. They offered a support system to facilitate the healing process confidentially in a safe place.

In the five years A Movement of Love has existed, we have used different ways to touch on the subject of abortion:

- **Education on Life Sunday**—Highlighting concrete scientific facts of the developing baby in the womb.
- **Sermons**—Taking a biblical perspective on ideas such as, "if it's legal, it's okay," and emphasizing that legalizing abortion does not

make the moral dilemma go away.

- **Skits**—Presenting a three-part skit called "Unthinkable," which portrays three stories of crisis pregnancy, abortion, and redemption after the abortion.
- **Men's voices**—Inviting guest male speakers to share their testimonies of abortion and forgiveness to the men's ministry group.
- **Informational nights**—Inviting women through the weekly event video to an informational night where they can hear stories from women who have gone through the healing process. Attendees are encouraged to go through the process themselves. Interactives work well during the information night, as women realize they can be heard and healed in the context of community.
- **Videos**—Posting videos on the church website that discuss abortion's effect on women and the opportunity to receive healing. The videos cover various topics and include testimonies from women who have gone through the healing process.

Step 4: Provide a place to heal

Church leaders should prayerfully consider adopting a study specifically designed for healing from abortion. My church offers a ten-week study called *Forgiven and Set Free* by Linda Cochrane, and there are several other quality resources available as well.

This is obviously a sensitive topic for people. Discretion and confidentiality are a must. Connecting people to the group leader or a facilitator is a way to help those who express interest in joining.

At our church, once a woman decides that she is indeed

interested, she completes a confidential in-take form, which is followed up by an interview. The purpose of the interview is to ensure that she is ready to go through the healing process and can commit to the entire ten to twelve weeks. Often this is the first time a woman is able to confide the secret of her abortion. No more than two weeks should transpire between the informational meeting and the beginning of the study.

Once the study begins, each participant signs a confidentiality agreement and a commitment for regular attendance. The meetings take place discreetly in a ministry room of the church, just like a Bible study or other ministry gathering. They last for ninety minutes, and childcare is provided. Many pregnancy centers offer these studies, but I find it powerful restorative justice when churches offer them.

I was honored to assist my pastor in co-leading the first study five years ago, and I am in awe of the transformative power healing brings to women through this ministry.

While there are things that women can do to begin processing their grief—seeking God and His intervention, connecting with things that bring them joy, consciously showing themselves grace, etc., I would like to stress the importance of seeking out a community with which to process the grief. Isolation can be a huge barrier to healing. When isolated, it is easy to fall prey to lies about who we are and what we are destined to be. There are many groups and resources available to women who want to find healing. Overcoming the grief of a traumatic event isn't about a quick fix. It takes dedication and people who will support those in the (sometimes long) process. With community also comes leadership experience and proven resources.

While several resources are listed within the appendices at the back of this book, I encourage inquiring at local churches to see if group ministries are available. It is important to note that these ministries take confidentiality seriously at every level, and women need not fear being shamed. No one has to know about their past and that they are seeking help.

I will be forever grateful to the ministry that helped Arica find healing and restore wholeness to her life. It took years for her to be at this place of rejuvenation, and my prayer is that other women don't have to wait so long. Her choice to share publicly exudes freedom. May this poem, written by Arica as an expression of her healing, minister to the hearts of those who have also walked this path.

"Acknowledge Me"

Please take a moment and stop.
Please take a moment and just be still.
Please… allow yourself to be real.

Allow yourself to feel.
Mommy, please listen.
It is time for you to heal.

There is something you must embrace.
I need you to imagine our gaze.
Do you perceive doting over my precious little face,
Drawing me in cheek to cheek,

Choose Zoe

Squeezing my bare, spongy feet?

Take hold of who I am.
My spirit is uniquely my own,
And I do not hide from being seen, named, or known.

Recognize that I did and still do exist.
I am yours and you are mine, this reality defies time.
Just give yourself a moment and allow it to sink in.

I was intricately woven together and perfectly placed within your
womb.
Although the days formed for me were few, my existence did not
cease.
Rest assured that our heavenly Father eagerly raptured me into
eternity.

So don't worry, Mom, do not shun away or feel ashamed.
Let today be the end of your denial and pain.

It pleases me to place this key into the palm of your hand.
It's for you to choose to take hold of this truth.
Can't you see that I live on through you?

Acknowledge me.
Allow the most perfect love to bring you inner peace.
I speak blessings over you.

The time has come to close this chapter of your book,
And to consciously choose to let yourself off the hook.

No more sadness, anger, or fear.
No more perfectionism or inability to allow me or others near.
No more grief, ridicule, unforgiveness, or blame can remain.

Death shall not consume either me or you,
Because the merciful love of our Father and His affection
overflows from my heart toward you.

Mommy, please dare to know,
I am at peace and abounding in love.
I am not alone or scared, and many others are here.

In great anticipation we joyfully await,
For the day we'll embrace our mothers as they enter heaven's
pearly gates.

Yes, you and I will be reunited again.
So it's time that you live knowing you are loved and forgiven.

Be free.
Free to acknowledge me.
Free to love.
Free to live.

Free to experience lasting joy and abundance.

You are free, Mommy.
Free to share hope.
Free to encourage others that it's true for them too.
You and I are the reconciled proof.

Beauty can be made from ashes, and mourning does turn into gladness.
Thank you, Mommy.
I'm so proud to see you fearlessly acknowledging me and accepting your release key.

With Eternal Love,

From Your Baby Above

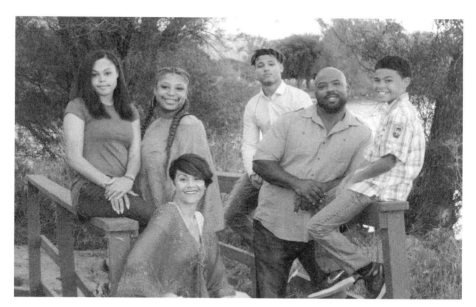

Arica's family

CHAPTER 9

If Only: Miscarriage and Infertility

It's his hands that stand out in my memory—his perfectly formed, tiny hands. The hands of my baby boy, born too soon. I was seventeen years old and pregnant…again.

"Wait," you say. "Didn't you learn your lesson after you got pregnant the first time?"

No. No, I did not. The glue of sex, meant to bond a man and woman for life, had bonded me to Arica's father. Dogged by my childhood molestation, and in the absence of any discussion surrounding sex and my pregnancy, I continued with what I knew. And what I knew was that I thought I was madly in love with this boy, sex made me feel wanted, and he would eventually dedicate himself to me and our growing family.

Bad decision begat bad decision, and I came to be twenty-two weeks pregnant, squatting miserably in my bathtub at three thirty in the morning. Having been through labor with Arica, I knew that was what was happening to me now. The pain from the contractions was intense. I desperately wanted my mother, but the bedrooms were adjacent to the bathroom, and I feared waking Arica or my dad. In a voice that was part sob, part silent scream, I called for her, but she couldn't hear me.

There was an extreme contraction, and something landed in the tub. That's when I saw him. My perfect little baby boy. His hands and feet were splayed, and I could tell he was no longer in the sac. He was the size of a small doll, probably just over a pound in weight.

I became paralyzed in motion and thought.

Though I wanted to resuscitate him, I didn't know how. In recent years, babies as young as twenty-two weeks have been known to survive outside the womb with specialized care, but this was the 1970s, and I was sitting in a bathtub with no idea what to do. I felt utterly helpless. My mind wandered. I thought of the story of Moses in the Bible and how helpless his mother must have felt as she placed him in the basket and sent him down the river.

It must have felt like this. I looked at my baby and said, "Moses. You are my Moses."

After about twenty minutes, my mom finally heard me and came in.

"Laura, are you okay?" she asked.

I turned my face into the flowered curtain and sobbed. I couldn't bear to look in the tub any longer.

"Laura, what's wrong? Are you…are you pregnant again?"

"Not anymore," I managed to say through the choking pain and tears.

"Oh, dear God. Get up," she said, her voice full of concern and compassion. My mom picked up Moses's delicate body—an exquisite miniature of his sister, Arica. As she cradled him, I could see those tiny, perfect hands.

"What are you going to do with him?" I asked.

"I'm going to take him to the hospital. You get cleaned up and put on a pad and go back to bed."

I watched her walk out of the bathroom holding my baby.

That night in the bathroom I was introduced to postpartum loss. In that moment, I joined the millions of women who lose babies every year to miscarriage. It is estimated that upwards of 20 percent of pregnancies end in miscarriage, most of which occur in the first trimester. But postpartum loss isn't reserved for miscarriage. It encompasses a host of situations: stillbirth, loss during childbirth or in the NICU, SIDS, and, as discussed previously, abortion. Though not technically postpartum loss, I would also include infertility and giving a baby up for adoption in this category. While there are obvious differences, I chose to group them here because all involve grief from either the loss of a physical child or the dream of a child.

People facing these situations need to know they are not alone. Many families are journeying through similar difficult times. And while some process through the stages of grief more quickly than others, these experiences are deeply personal. No one has the right to tell those in this situation how to feel or how they should be healing. The path through grief for any reason is often a marathon, not a sprint, and postpartum loss is no exception. No one needs to hear that she or he should be getting over the loss in a more timely manner.

Muddling through the stages of grief often involves drastic mood shifts that are normal. For a woman who is also experiencing altered brain chemistry from the major hormonal effects of a pregnancy, these shifts can be exacerbated and much more difficult to comprehend or contain. Partners and loved ones need to be sensitive to these drastic changes and acknowledge that the physical effects of the loss will have a greater impact on the woman.

While the time spent in the varying stages of grief may be long, it is important not to assume the cause is depression. Grief just takes time. That being said, if someone feels stuck in a particular stage of grief, especially if that stage is debilitating, it may be a sign of clinical depression. Seeking the help of a Christian counselor or therapist may be needed. One never needs to be ashamed for seeking help. Being humble and courageous enough to admit the need for help is a sign of strength, not weakness. This is true in the case of depression and the need for guidance in navigating the changes postpartum loss has wrought in relationships.

Couples experiencing pregnancy loss or infertility often have to find new ways to relate to each other. For some, tragedy creates an increased fear of loss and may cause a person to cling more tightly to the things she or he loves, even to the extent of codependence. Others may feel the need to isolate themselves. Each may be processing the loss differently, and the assumption on the part of one partner that the other should be further along in the grief cycle can be damaging to a relationship and the capacity for trust in years to come. All of these responses are normal, but they can be confusing and difficult to navigate and must be handled with care. Along with love, grace, openness, and patience, assistance from a trained professional can be of tremendous help to families.

Sometimes one of the more difficult aspects of dealing with loss is, frankly, dealing with other people. Some people seem to naturally know what to say and do, while others just stick their feet in their mouths or ignore the situation altogether. We've all heard stories of people saying tremendously insensitive things:

"Don't worry, you can still have another baby."
"At least you hadn't done the nursery yet."
"Now you can drink again."
"There was probably something wrong with it."
"Aren't you over that yet?"

The list could go on, but the point is made: Some people are bad at this. To be fair, most people want to be helpful and supportive during a time of loss but just don't know how to be or what to say. Society has taught us either to avoid difficult things or to fix them. But neither of these approaches works with grief. People enduring loss need to have their pain acknowledged, but they don't need to be told how to fix it or why it isn't as bad as they thought. What they need to know is that someone is there. Someone is listening. Someone cares. It could be as simple as saying, "I'm so sorry this happened. I'm here if you ever want to talk." Compassion can further be demonstrated by offering to run errands or bring dinner. If the person in pain is too polite to accept, another way to approach it is to say, "I've made a freezer meal for you. When can I drop it by?"

If men and women suffering loss do choose to open up, it is vital that those to whom they choose to open up don't judge them for their feelings and don't rush them through their grief. Being surrounded by someone else's pain might be uncomfortable, but fight the urge to pull away. Instead, be there for the long haul. When weeks turn into months, continue to show support. While life continues for those around them, people dealing with loss may feel like theirs has come to a standstill. Once they feel it is no longer acceptable to voice their grief, they will internalize it, leading others to believe they are over it, when in truth they are still suffering. Don't be the reason someone else feels they should stuff their grief.

Conversely, for the families suffering postpartum loss, it will be natural to connect with people who are supportive and allow space for grief. Relationships may change. Friends who were close and enjoyable pre-loss may seem distant, unsupportive, or even hurtful. It is okay to let those friendships fade. One should not feel guilty pursuing relationships that are life-giving during this difficult time. It can be especially helpful to find those who have had similar experiences and who can better understand the heartache. If interactions prove difficult with loved ones with whom distancing is neither practical nor wanted, some families have found it helpful to write an open letter, detailing their feelings, their expectations of interaction, and what they find to be helpful and hurtful. This can remove the guesswork for loved ones and may very well save relationships.

All of this was illustrated in my own life. The night of my miscarriage, I did as I was told. In a daze, I walked back to my room, glancing at the plaque on the door that had a pink princess announcing my name. I felt far from being a princess in that moment. I crawled into bed with my disappointment, pulled the yellow-flowered sheets over my head, and wept myself to sleep.

The next morning, my mother took me first thing to the doctor for a follow-up, and that was the last we spoke of it for twenty-five years. I assumed Moses was already dead when she left with him the night before and that she had likely taken him to the hospital or to our family friends who owned the funeral home. Being good Catholics, it was the practice to always properly bury the dead, no matter how small. Miscarried babies were given an appropriate burial, whether added to another casket or given their own.

My mom told my dad I wasn't feeling well and that the two of them would be taking Arica out of town for the day. She called my sister Mary and asked if she and my brother-in-law could come and sit with me. I didn't care who was there—I only wanted Moses.

We were in the kitchen when my milk came in. My baby was dead; why did my body have to cruelly remind me? Didn't it know there was no longer a baby who would need to nurse? I tried to ignore it. I remember sitting at the table—Mary and Charles across from me, completely unaware of my situation and playing dominoes—numb in my grief, replaying the events that transpired in my bathroom.

I thought back to three years earlier, sitting by the same tub, as my dog, Mimi, had tried to bring life into this world, only to have it ripped away from her. I had gone against my parents' wishes and bred her with a dog down the street. She was too old to go through a pregnancy, but I had really wanted puppies and thought it surely wouldn't be as bad as my parents had said. She had her puppies in our bathtub, but none of them survived, and I was powerless to save them. Mimi, meanwhile, tore at the doggy bed and whimpered and howled in misery. I knew what happened to Mimi in that bathtub was my fault, and now I was certain what happened there last night was my fault as well.

Twelve hours before I had glimpsed my baby boy for the first and last time, I had seen his father at the park...rolling around in the grass with a new girl who had just arrived from Chicago. He had driven me to school that morning and was supposed to be driving me home. I hadn't seen his car, so I went looking for him in the park adjacent to my school in case he had arrived early and was killing time. Killing time, indeed.

Blinding rage and hurt welled up within me. Thoughts swirled through my head. This boy was the father of my baby girl, who at this very moment was waiting for me to get home from school. I was carrying his second child, and we all know how I had come to be pregnant. History proved that he had a hard time being faithful, but just the night before, he held me in his arms and told me he loved me.

I wanted to scream, *Who do you think you are? How could you? Did you forget about our child? Are you a monster? What does this tramp have that I don't?* Instead, the only thing that came out of my mouth was, "What are you doing?"

Chapter 9

He stopped getting to know the new girl. He glanced up at me and then back down at Miss Chicago.

"I'm not with her," he said, gesturing in my general direction.

I was no longer at a loss for words. "Not with *me*? Are you crazy? What are you talking about? You were with me last night!"

He had officially poked the bear, and he knew it. He got up and began to back away from me as I continued to berate him. The anger that had been building inside exploded through my fists. I began to physically lash out at him, and he defended himself, moving out of reach of my arms and legs. We continued in this manner across the entire expanse of the park and two blocks into the residential area.

Hell truly hath no fury like a woman scorned.

In a moment of sheer ferocity, my hands made contact, and I shoved him with all my strength. He stumbled and fell, but as he did so, his legs flew into the air, and his knee landed squarely in my stomach. It's a feeling and a moment I'll never forget.

Physically and emotionally exhausted, I left him there. I don't even remember how I got home, but somehow I managed. Arica was there waiting for me, her sweet, chubby baby hands grabbing my fingers and patting my face. I felt disconnected, but she brought me back to reality. I took care of her as I usually did, had dinner, then went to bed early. I didn't feel well. Later that night, lying alone in my bed, the contractions started, and that's how I ended up in the bathtub.

I could not stop blaming myself for my son's death. If only I hadn't gotten into a fight. If only I hadn't pushed my boyfriend. If only I had seen my self-worth and decided that I and my babies deserved better and had just walked away. If only I'd taught him to treat me better by not going along with his cheating when it had happened before. If only I'd listened to my parents and never gotten involved with a boy who didn't believe what I did in the first place.

If only, if only, if only.

The "if only" game is a common one for women who have experienced postpartum loss. When misery and pain come at us, we naturally try to find someone or something to blame. Often, we ultimately settle on ourselves. Some women blame their bodies for their incapacity to house or sustain life, disregarding the reality that it could be genetic factors for which they or their partner have no control. If a woman experiences increased infertility because of a previous D&C, her guilt may be even higher. Others, like me, live in guilt for the choices that led to the circumstances surrounding our pregnancy loss. We even feel guilt for getting through our grief, because we think it means we are forgetting our loss and the person it represents. It's a vicious circle.

Whatever the situation surrounding our guilt, we can't begin to heal until we let it go. Whether through forgiveness for our actions, acceptance of our bodies, or realization that healing does not equate with forgetting, we must accept the grace God freely offers for our lives. For the things we can change about our situation, He can give us the power and will to make those changes. He can also give us the courage to face the things over which we have no control. Either way, we are not alone and we are not helpless.

Postpartum loss can also be particularly difficult because it is often a hidden grief. A mom with a child on her hip clearly has the public identity of being a mother. This is not the case for those who have lost their children. The outside world does not see the motherhood that was lost and the way it shapes identity. In many cases, very few outside people, if any, knew of the pregnancy to begin with. This can leave a woman or couple feeling isolated in their grief. For those struggling with infertility, this may be especially true. In a culture of few boundaries, people often feel free to ask about parenthood plans. Couples dealing with infertility are subjected to well-meaning but insensitive questions about when they plan to start a family or why it is taking so long. Many couples are not open about their infertility, and thus childbearing ability cannot be assumed. I find it a good practice to just not ask and therefore not risk the chance of unknowingly causing pain. If someone wants to talk to me about when or if she plans to have children, she will do so without my asking.

Because couples tend not to broadcast their infertility, many don't realize its prevalence. According to infertility specialist Dr. Royster, 10–15 percent of all couples in the United States struggle with some sort of infertility.[66] Of those, 85 percent are caused by three main reasons. First, a woman may not be ovulating properly due to a variety of factors, such as age, an endocrine imbalance, or being overweight. Secondly, a woman may have an anatomical issue, such as fibroids or scar tissue. Finally, one third of infertility issues are the result of a male factor, such as low sperm count or mobility of the sperm. Couples dealing with infertility may have a particularly difficult time not blaming themselves or their biology for their inability to conceive, but Dr. Royster is quick to remind them that their biology is not their fault.

Modern medicine offers many possible solutions for infertility, but it isn't a fail-safe. While some issues, such as a blocked fallopian tube, are relatively simple to treat, high maternal age or uterine scarring, often caused by abortion or other medical procedures, can be more difficult. Couples seeking infertility treatment have generally invested a great deal of time and finances in the process. This can become a consuming part of their lives, and loved ones need to realize and respect the physical and emotional toll it can take.

Dr. Royster also notes the importance partner involvement plays in the process. Infertility diagnosis and treatments can be emotional and daunting and are lengthy processes. His heart breaks for the women who go through it unsupported. While he can't speak to statistics, anecdotally, he sees a huge difference in the emotional stability of women who have available partners who come with them to multiple appointments versus men who show up only when the sperm is needed. As a husband and father of daughters, he would hate to have a loved one go through that by herself.

Couples wrestling with infertility might look at a teen mom like I was, who couldn't seem to help getting pregnant, and feel anger or confusion. How is it fair that there are women getting pregnant who don't even want babies? It is a valid question, one for which I don't know the answer. And while one cannot blame the woman who easily conceives for that blessing, one also cannot blame the couples encountering infertility for having negative emotional reactions at the sight of it.

Having feelings of loss triggered by various scenes of parenthood is normal. Reactions may occur when least expected or be provoked by something that seems totally unrelated. For me, I was reminded of the pain when I saw flowered curtains that looked like the one in my parents' bathroom. It isn't meant to feel offensive or personal when a grieving couple feels sadness at the sight of a baby or pregnant woman or needs to bow out of a baby shower here or there. It is simply a manifestation of their grief and does not mean they don't value or feel joy for the new parents. People can rejoice at new life being formed in someone else, while at the same time mourning their inability to do the same. It is not mutually exclusive—sorrow can live with gratitude.

My dear friend Janice knows this well. Having struggled with infertility for years while fostering children, Janice and her husband were given the gift of their daughter when one brave woman chose to carry her unplanned pregnancy to term and give her daughter up for adoption. When their adopted daughter, Jenna, came into their lives, Janice dutifully packaged up the pain of her infertility and buried it deep. She thought that remembering the disappointment over their infertility seemed a betrayal to the blessing of their daughter. When her husband would bring up his desire for a biological child or the possibility of finding a solution to infertility, she would remind him of his need to be grateful for the baby they had. After continuous rebuffing of his angst, he eventually quit mentioning it. Looking back, Janice can see how her dismissive attitude about his feelings may have led him not to share other vulnerable parts of himself with her. She denied their marriage the gift of grieving together, therefore denying them the chance to grow in intimacy.[67]

It wasn't until recently—more than twenty years after Jenna's adoption—that God showed her how deeply she had buried her dream of having biological children and how stuffing those feelings, and forcing her husband to do the same, denied one of the truths Jesus offers through the zoe life: that pain and beauty, loss and gain, can coexist. Much like the simultaneous sense of loss and gratitude felt when a loved one who has suffered from a prolonged illness finally receives a pain-free life in heaven, so can the feelings be of those who have adopted in the midst of infertility.

"Why now, God, after all these years?" Janice wondered.

"Because I want you in joy to live the rest of your life, and *enjoy* the rest of your life," she heard God answer.

Once God brought her neglected grief to the surface, Janice was able to truly mourn the loss of her dream for biological children. With the help of a counselor in her church, Janice first worked through her own grief, and then she approached her husband and asked his forgiveness for denying him expression of his. What has transpired is a renewed trust within their marriage and a deeper understanding of the fullness of the zoe life.

I understand Janice's consternation at healing coming after so many years, because it was much the same for me. My healing began in an unlikely place: with two rivers—one in Montana and the other in Honduras—nearly three decades after my miscarriage.

Shortly before my mom died, we were together, and she mentioned someone losing a baby. In that moment, I gathered the courage to ask the question I had wanted to ask for more than twenty-five years.

"Mom, what did you do with my baby?"

I could! tell the question caught her off guard. She paused for a moment, staring off into the distance, as if watching a distant memory play out before her eyes. Then she slowly said, "Laura, I took him to the Yellowstone River. I blessed him, and I baptized him, and then...I put him in a jar and sent him down the river."

She looked at me, and we both had tears in our eyes. I couldn't believe what I had just heard. For a moment I was shocked. I trusted her, but it seemed cold and harsh to think of my baby careening down a wild river alone at the mercy of raw nature.

A few years after my mom told me about her experience with Moses in the Yellowstone, I had my own experience in a river. My eldest brother had made a promise to my mother before she died that all the siblings would get together every year. One brother and his wife were missionaries in Honduras, so we all decided to meet there that year. Someone had the bright idea to go white water rafting. The river was insane. We all took turns thinking we were going to die—seriously. I wouldn't have guessed at the beginning of the excursion that the river would save my life instead.

At one point, I fell into the turbulent water. Waves were crashing over my head, and I felt my body being pulled along as if I were powerless. I couldn't get out of the water.

The guide threw a rope to me, and my brother was yelling, "Swim! Swim! You have to swim, Squirt!"

"I can't!" I screamed, feeling panicked. I honestly thought I was going to drown.

And then...

And then God, as He has mercifully done so many times in my life, ruled over my chaos. His Spirit calmed the waters in my head, and it hit me: *I lost my baby, and he was left in a river. Now I am in a river.* It was the first time I had been in a river since I had learned of the Yellowstone experience, and the connection of the two rivers overwhelmed me. I began to weep. My family must have thought I was crying from fear, but I wasn't thinking about that anymore. For the very first time, I was examining a grief that I had buried for thirty years.

"God," I sobbed, "the grief is too much! I lost my baby! *He was left in a river!* What did you have for him at the end of that river?"

In my heart I heard the reply, "He came into my arms." I had been shocked when my mother told me about the Yellowstone story, but now a different image came to mind. Whether she knew it or not, by taking him to the river, she was reenacting one of the most powerful scenes in biblical history, the rescue of Moses on the Nile. But this time instead of Pharaoh's daughter finding a helpless, squalling babe, my lifeless Moses would be floating down into the arms of my Father in heaven. My son had a personal service with his grandmother and then had been lovingly sent down the river. I thought I was the only one who knew his name, but at that moment I was reminded that God had known his name. He had given my mother the inclination to care for my baby by placing him in that river, just as He had cared for Moses long ago. A tremendous peace washed over me.

It broke me and restored me at the same time. That was what I wanted to do! I wanted to go into His arms. I began swimming furiously, repeating, "I can do all things through Christ who strengthens me."

Clearly, I didn't die. But the need to reject my grief did. When we got to the end of the river, all I could think about was being baptized. I had been a Christian for years, but never made it a point to be baptized. Now the desire permeated me to the core of my being. So baptized I was, in a river in Honduras made a little fuller by my tears. No one understood the significance of that river but me, and it felt like God and I were sharing a private, personal moment like my mom had shared with Moses. He was offering to bring beauty out of my mess, joy out of my pain, and I humbly accepted.

The healing process that began in Honduras continued for several years. With the help of a study on healing from miscarriage offered through Alpha Pregnancy Clinics, I worked through my grief and pain. One of the hardest things to let go of was the guilt. Reading Kathe Wunnenberg's *Grieving the Child I Never Knew* helped me immensely. It showed me that I was punishing myself by looking at the past to see where I could have changed things and letting guilt push me away from God instead of toward Him.

It was a difficult process, but I have finally been able to release that to God and receive His acceptance of me. The love of God and family helped me to endure. I know that moving on with my life does not equate with forgetting Moses or dishonoring his memory. I will always remember and love my child, but that memory no longer threatens to hold me back from the zoe life. The loss of Moses is part of what makes me who I am, and I look forward to the day we sit under the Tree of Zoe together.

CHAPTER 10

Adoption: A Courageous Sacrifice

As far back as he can remember, Dillon has loved baseball. Wherever he went, he was playing the game in his mind even if he didn't have equipment handy. He would pretend to strike people out in the grocery store and swing a home run in the parking lot. When he did have a ball and glove in reach, he'd head for the closest curb and throw the ball at just the right spot so it would come shooting back at him and he could practice infield drills. If a fence was nearby, he'd chuck the ball over and try to jump the fence and catch it just like an outfielder robbing a home run. He spent as much time outside as he could. He felt good out there. This was his escape from the terror of his childhood. Outside there was no screaming. Outside the hands manipulated by drugs didn't touch him.[68]

Inside, well now, that was a different story. Inside his mom was coping with debilitating pain. At some point before Dillon's memories began to take root, she had slipped in a puddle of water in a grocery store—caused by a broken vase—and broke her back. For a time, she heavily medicated with prescription drugs, but eventually the doctor stopped prescribing them. That's when she turned to other drugs to ease the pain. Some days she could hold herself together better than others, and on those days, she almost seemed like a functional parent, picking him up from daycare and kindergarten. But she was always late. Though he was young, he remembers the humiliation of waiting with the childcare staff long after the other kids had gone home, for his mom to remember to come and get him.

Those were the good days. The bad days were the ones when they would physically assault each other, and she would chase him around the apartment with a pair of scissors or a butcher knife. The neighbors would complain about the noise, and the police were called, but nothing ever really changed. Eventually, every day became a bad day. The police grew annoyed at their repeated visits, and the neighbors became weary of their disturbances, so Dillon and his mom were kicked out of their apartment and began a nomadic life.

Dillon's dad had partial custody, and Dillon would spend time at his place as well, always having to wait at the police station for the swap because his parents couldn't stand to see each other. He doesn't have a lot of memories of his dad, but one is crystal clear. They were driving on the freeway, Dillon sitting up front with his dad, gazing out the window at the California landscape.

"Hey, kid," his dad said. "You want to see a match burn twice?"

"All right, I guess," Dillon replied.

His dad pulled out a matchbook, the kind he picked up at a bar or hotel lobby somewhere. Letting go of the steering wheel, he tore off a match and expertly lit it. Then he blew it out. Dillon was disappointed. That trick wasn't cool at all.

"Let me see your wrist," his dad directed.

Dillon pushed his wrist over to the driver's side, and his dad imbedded the still glowing match into it. He yelped in pain. Terrified, he jumped into the back seat and tried to hide. Up front, his dad chuckled. Dillon was six years old.

Dillon never told his mom about the burn, but she found out through one of his friends. Shortly after that, she was awarded full custody. Not having to spend any more time with his father was good, but being with his mom full time was not. Her drug use was increasing, and so was the conflict and the abuse.

When he reached first grade, he made fast friends with a little boy who asked him to spend the night. He liked his friend's house, and before long, Dillon's mom was encouraging him to stay there more and more. He isn't sure at what point he realized it was really a group home and that his mom had been manipulating the situation for him to live there all along, but the reality wounded him deeply. Looking back, he knows his mom was trying to do what was best for him, but it is hard to separate that from the feeling of rejection.

His mom went into rehabilitation, and he went to live with a foster family. The expectation was that she would get clean in six months and the two would be reunited. That never happened. Just before she was to graduate from the program, she and Dillon had a great visit at a park, where they played in the sand and on a swing set. As they said their goodbyes, a motorcycle roared up. Dillon's dad appeared on the scene and brought her drugs. Her graduation was sabotaged, and her son's dreams of reunification annihilated. In his mind, she had chosen drugs and a tenuous relationship with his dad over him. Her parental rights were terminated, and Dillon was put up for adoption.

Adoption. The word conjures up a variety of emotions based on experience and perspective. Some, like Dillon, encounter adoption at an age when they remember the trauma of the process, while others are adopted as infants and it is all they have ever known. To a mother who has placed her child for adoption, the word might carry a certain amount of consolation, knowing she put her child's welfare first, but there may also be a sense of loss. Conversely, an adoptive parent hearing the word may feel overwhelming joy and gratitude. I acknowledge that the topic is complex and that there are tales of horror, for which my heart breaks. But far outnumbering the tragedies are the beautiful stories—lives forever changed by the miracle of strangers becoming family.

I believe placing a baby for adoption when it is better for the child is one of the most noble acts a person can commit. It is the essence of allowing beauty to flourish out of chaos. As a mother, having carried my babies in my body and then having the privilege of raising them, it is hard for me to fathom the level of love, courage, and selflessness needed for this act. It leaves me breathless.

Every adoptive parent I have spoken to will corroborate these feelings. For many, adoption made the long-held dream of parenthood a reality. It is estimated that, on average, there are thirty-six couples waiting to adopt for every one child placed for adoption.[69] While it is my hope that every parent who desires to raise his or her child would find the resources and support to do so, it is also clear that, for those who decide parenting their child isn't an option, there is no shortage of people who would cherish the opportunity to do it on their behalf. It can be difficult for adoptive parents to express the level of emotion and gratitude they feel for the privilege of adopting, but one adoptive mother says it beautifully:

> *My heart is bursting with both love for my son and gratitude to the woman who gave me this gift of a child. I don't know if I would have had the courage to make that sacrifice. As an adoptive mother, I grieve for his birth mother. Because I love my son so dearly, I cannot imagine the grief of living without him, and I hurt for her. I esteem her greatly for being brave in the face of such loss. She remained focused on what she believed was best for her child despite the pain of her own loss in the process. She continues to choose to focus on how she and her child found love in a hopeless place. She is a living example of how choosing life and adoption supports what we believe about God's never-failing love: He chooses us, sacrifices everything for us, and adopts us as His own.[70]*

When considering adoption, women and men can make decisions both they and potential adoptive parents can live with. Birth parents who can't commit to raising a child but wrestle with the notion of losing all contact *can* stipulate that they want an open adoption.

Adoption agencies can facilitate an understanding between birth and adoptive parents regarding the expectations for involvement and contact.

In addition to specifying an open adoption, parents voluntarily giving their children up for adoption have access to in-depth profiles on prospective adoptive parents. While it may be tempting to choose parents based on financial status, many birth parents note the importance of going deeper. What does their family history say about the kind of parents they will be? Assuming the child has a temperament similar to the birth parents, do the prospective parents have the qualities needed to nurture such a temperament? If an open adoption is desired, does their profile and the early interactions indicate they will work to make it happen? Finding parents that exhibit these tendencies can relieve some of the anxiety felt by birth parents.

This process proved true for one woman named Marta and eased her fear. Over eight months pregnant and convinced she could barely care for the two children she already had, let alone this new baby, she sought help for an adoption. Having looked over the list of prospective adoptive parents in her area, she settled on a couple who exhibited the life and history she thought would be worthy of her daughter. Marta asked them to attend her first—and only, it turns out—prenatal screening. That was how she met Janice and Alan. Remember my friend Janice who stuffed her grief over infertility for over two decades? This was the beginning of her dream of parenthood being realized. Five days after they met Marta, Jenna entered both of their worlds. As much as Marta loved her baby, she made the difficult and courageous decision to carry through with the adoption.[71]

Marta felt constant contact would be too difficult, both for her and Jenna, and asked that Janice not allow Jenna to contact her until she turned eighteen. As she was growing up, the absence of relationship proved difficult at times for Jenna. Thankfully, Janice says, when it came to grief, she took a different approach with their daughter than she had with herself and her husband. While Janice had thought it dishonoring to feel the loss of infertility after adopting Jenna, she encouraged her daughter to fully embrace the coexistence of grief and joy in her own life. Janice knew that allowing Jenna to feel and talk about the loss of her birthmother in no way diminished the love for them, her adoptive parents. If anything, it made their relationship stronger. While Janice and Alan told Jenna she was adopted from the beginning, and even had a picture in the baby album of her birthmother holding her, it wasn't until Jenna was five years old that she spoke about it directly.

The family was fostering two older children, who, to this day, are considered part of their family. Jenna's foster sister was going through a difficult time not being with her mother and had been frequently voicing her displeasure. Jenna was sitting in a chair in the bathroom while Janice did her hair. Looking at her mother's reflection in the mirror, Jenna took Janice by surprise when she asked, "Well, how come I can't be with my *real* mom? It makes me so mad!"

Any parent might feel a twinge of rejection at those words or try to soothe the child by convincing her she should not be sad because she had a family who loved her. While Janice felt all those things, she also felt wisdom from God flowing through her.

"It makes me mad too, sweetheart! God's original design was for you to be with your birth mommy and daddy and for your [foster] sister to be with her birth parents too. But that didn't happen for many reasons, and it is okay to be sad about it. I'm glad God chose us to be your adoptive family."

"Oh," Jenna said before playing with her hair ribbons again, seemingly satisfied.

That was not the last time the subject of Jenna's birthmother came up, but every time it did, her parents encouraged her to feel what she needed to feel and assured her that they weren't threatened by any of it. Though she showed interest in finding her birth mother throughout her teen years, when Jenna turned eighteen, she grew hesitant. A few months after her birthday, she received a message on social media from a girl who said she believed they were sisters. It was just the nudge she needed. Her parents helped her confirm the information, and one sunny day, with their blessing, Jenna took a friend and met her birth family at a park. Today, Jenna is a thriving adult whose renewed relationship with her birth family has enriched all of their lives. Janice's confession to her about her own denial of loss in the presence of gain has given Jenna continued freedom to emotionally process what it means to be adopted. Janice and Alan are closer than ever with their daughter and marvel at the way her relationship with her birth family has further spread the gospel and the realization of a zoe life.

Permission to grieve the loss of a birth family, while not threatening the feelings of an adoptive family, is something many adopted children wish they possessed. In a survey conducted for this book, adults who were adopted as children consistently stated this was the thing they most desired to have changed about their childhood; this also applied to their current experiences as adults in relation to their adoptive families.[72] They longed for the freedom to discuss their birth family and the circumstances surrounding their adoptions with their adoptive parents.

Some families are wonderfully open on this topic, while others shy away from it. Whether from insecurity on the parents' part or a desire to make children feel that they were not different from other members of the family, many parents never openly discussed the circumstances of their child's adoption in any depth or the feelings related to it. This lack of discourse often implicitly made the children feel like it was not a subject to be broached, and so they never did, even though they had a tremendous desire to do so. While unintended, this led to some of those children feeling a certain amount of isolation from the adoptive family. They appreciated that their parents wanted to make them feel "just like one of the family," but denying a huge part of their identity—their adoption—had the opposite effect. They wished their parents truly understood that curiosity about or even pain felt from losing their birth family was not a reflection of diminished love and devotion to the adoptive family.

The inherent loss felt by many adoptive children is what advocate Sophia Cruz describes as a "soul wound." After traumatic circumstances surrounding her pregnancy and birth of her son, Sophia did her best to raise him though she was only fifteen. But after a year, extenuating circumstances led her to place him for adoption for his own safety. The decision was excruciating, but she felt it was the only viable option. Despite her personal tragedies, Sophia never gave up. She built a good and safe life for herself and a second child, whom she was able to raise. Now she advocates for parents on both sides of an adoption to acknowledge this soul wound in children and to provide the security and permission to address it. No matter how secure or loved children are in their adoptive family, they will always feel an emotional and genetic connection to their biological parents on some level. Sophia asserts that to deny this connection and to negatively view the duality that can exist in loving two sets of parents only harms the child.[73] For example, if children express sadness over separation or loss of relationship with biological parents, it isn't especially helpful to tell them how loved they are by their adoptive parents. Those reactions only serve to invalidate their feelings when what they hope for is to be understood and not to feel like they are disappointing adoptive families. Their sadness is not about feeling unloved by the adoptive parents; it really isn't about the adoptive parents at all. Children can feel secure in their love of their adoptive families and still feel the very deep soul wound of losing their biological ones.

Whenever possible, allowing children to have some sort of connection to their biological family can be healing. This can be difficult for both the adoptive and birth parents for many reasons. What I hear most frequently, assuming birth parents are in a stable place capable of relationship, is that adoptive parents may feel threatened and worry that, despite having raised them, their children might grow to love their birth parents more, especially since they have the genetic connection. Birth parents may feel that the close connection will be too painful and a constant reminder of what they gave up or of a difficult period in their lives.

When asked about this complex and delicate balance, Sophia emphasizes that what both sides need to remember is that it really isn't about the parents. At its core, parenting with unconditional love is really about the child and what is best for him or her. Fears, anxiety, and insecurity must be set aside for the good of the children. Does that mean all boundaries are tossed aside and children are thrown into situations where they could be traumatized or harmed? Absolutely not; a child's physical, spiritual, and emotional well-being must always be paramount. What it does mean, however, is that adults must work through their own insecurities and issues in order to discuss and, hopefully, facilitate relationships that heal the child's soul wound, even if it is uncomfortable for the parents. Sophia reiterates that if birth parents are safe and stable, allowing them to be an additional source of love for the child can only make the child feel more loved. Parents who practice true unconditional love will instill the knowledge in their children that they will support whatever is best for them and that nothing will affect status in the family. Parents who aren't threatened are a gift to their children. By promoting healing, parents help their children tap into the zoe life.

Many adoptive parents understand the value in their children having a relationship with their birth family. But what can they do when the birth family isn't interested? It is not uncommon for birth parents to indicate a desire for an open adoption, but either back out or taper off. This trend makes sense when one considers that many birth parents are young and still figuring out their place in life. Careers, new relationships, and new children can make maintaining these relationships complex. Such is the case for one adoptive mom who discussed the challenges this presents in her own family. She has two children, one of whom has an active relationship with his birth family. The birth family of her other child, though initially in favor of an open adoption, later decided they would not like any contact. This has proved understandably painful for both mother and daughter, as the daughter observes her brother engaging in something she does not have. Though far from ideal, this wise mother uses this experience to validate her child's feelings of loss and create an atmosphere of stability and acceptance.

While acknowledgement of the soul wound of adoption was paramount with the adults surveyed, the survey prominently revealed a second issue of high importance: the desire for some sort of family history. Medically speaking, this makes common sense. Adoptive children, and by extension, their children, are often denied knowledge of their own medical history. This proves troubling when diagnosing illnesses that may be genetic as well as knowing when to be proactive about possible inherited traits. Think of all the forms and medical histories required at every medical appointment. I think I may have had to fill one out at a nail salon recently. I'm kidding about that, but they do seem endless. Now imagine having absolutely no idea about the answers to any of those questions. I think it would be nerve-wracking at best and terrifying at worst.

One survey respondent suffers from a disability acquired during infancy. The cause of this disability is often genetic, and if known, can be treated and possibly reduced. Had her adoptive parents been given a medical history, her life today could be very different.

But it isn't solely medical histories longed for by those who have been adopted. One respondent poignantly remembers sitting in a science class during a project on genetics. As her peers discussed the traits they received from their parents and grandparents, she sat staring at her blank paper, feeling utterly alone. Another respondent was in a history class where students gave reports on their ancestral heritage. She used her adoptive family's story, but it did not feel like her own. While both very much felt loved and cherished by their adoptive families, these instances made them keenly feel what one calls her "history-less-ness."

"I would have given anything," she said, "to have some sort of generic history of my biological family. I wouldn't have needed details that would invade privacy or reduce anonymity, but enough to give me a sense of where I came from." Were they immigrants? Does musical ability run in the family? Did they identify with a culture different from her adoptive family? What color eyes did they have? Anything would have been helpful and given her a sense of identity.

She went on to note that cultural background is often celebrated and nurtured in international adoptions, but it tends to be hidden or forgotten in domestic ones. If she could speak to mothers placing their children for adoption, her one piece of advice would be to consider giving both a medical history and some sort of redacted familial history to the adoptive family. If she could speak to adoptive parents, it would be to help their children find out what they could about their heritage. Little may be known about an adoptive child's ethnic or cultural background. With modern genetic testing, however, families can tap into data unavailable to previous generations. Perhaps that is an option to some families. Regardless of what information a family starts with, the sheer act of helping children discover what can be found of their cultural background will speak volumes. It communicates that unique cultural heritage is accepted, celebrated, important, and non-threatening. It is a tangible way to reassure children that the duality of feeling loss and gain, and even love for two sets of parents, is natural and welcomed.

The loss of identity can be particularly hard for children who have been adopted at an older age, as they already have an established identity with their birth family or have been denied an established identity by the nature of the foster system. The expectation that they will assume the identity of a new family can be confusing and challenging. This complexity is compounded by the fact that, while selecting parents for a young child in an adoption is often the prerogative of the birth parents or family services system, in situations like Dillon's, an older child has a measure of choice.

After a year and a half in a stable foster home, at the age of ten, Dillon was adopted by a different family. He planned to be adopted by young, rich city dwellers. Instead, what he got was an older middle class couple "who lived in the sticks," as he describes it. Having spent time with Mark and Vickie, Dillon knew he liked them, but when asked at his adoption hearing if he wanted to be adopted by them, he almost said no. They were nothing like the people he had imagined choosing. Still, standing there with everyone watching, he felt an unspoken pressure to say yes. So, he did. Up to that point, it was the best decision he had ever made.

Vickie and Mark had a choice too. Vickie experienced love at first sight when she saw Dillon. "It was spiritual," she says. In the same way, we are chosen through adoption into God's family. Consider this spiritual blessing in Ephesians 1:

> *Blessed be the God and Father of our Lord Jesus Christ, who has blessed us in Christ with every spiritual blessing in the heavenly places, even as he chose us in him before the foundation of the world, that we should be holy and blameless before him. In love he predestined us for adoption to himself as sons through Jesus Christ, according to the purpose of his will...*[74]

Still, it was anything but smooth sailing. They had done their research, and Dillon was convinced they had read all the parenting books on setting limits. He was their only child, and they could devote all their parental energies on him. He wasn't used to all the attention and expectations. There had never been any rules or consequences with his birth mom. Secretly, he loved that he finally had some boundaries in his life and people who cared enough to enforce them.

The problem was his rage. Years of being abused and lied to by the people he loved and trusted had wrapped his heart tightly with a layer of hurt so thick that he didn't know how to let love in. He was sure his adoptive parents would quit on him just like everyone else in his life, and he'd rather find out sooner than later. Whatever he could do to hurt them, he tried. He had been burned twice and would not be charmed a third time.

When he first arrived, he tried grabbing Vickie when he was angry with her, but soon found out that, in a house where men respected women, that would not be tolerated. So, he resorted to barricading himself in his room and screaming profanity and anything else he could think of to hurt them. When he was feeling particularly vindictive, he would threaten to poison the dogs.

Despite all his meanness, they proved him wrong. While they showed pain at his attempts to hurt them—and continued to set boundaries, Mark and Vickie never gave up on him. They stuck together and showed him love, through it all. And it was the showing that he really needed. People had *told* him things his whole life, but it was never backed up with action. His new dad didn't have to tell him anything—he showed by example, always. That spoke volumes, as did his new mother's generosity. He'd never had someone be so devoted to him. It felt strange at first, but it was attention he had craved. For the first time, he felt like he was really part of a family.

"It takes a real man to take in another man's child and love him like he is his own. That's what my dad did. He and my mom changed everything for me," he says with tears in his eyes.

If Dillon could speak to people considering adoption of older children, he would encourage them to really know what they are getting into. The road can be long and hard, and many of the children in that situation are dealing with severe trauma that can manifest in some pretty ugly ways, as his adoptive parents will tell you. He thinks prospective adoptive parents should be absolutely certain in their resolve before they try, because if the adoption doesn't work, there could be a child with even more trauma and scarring as a result.

If people are set in their resolve, the second thing he would tell them is to not to give up. "These kids really want to be loved and belong, even if their actions tell you otherwise. Be patient. Please, don't give up."

And what would he tell birth parents? "Your kids think about you as much as you think about them. You aren't forgotten. If you have a chance to reconcile, own up to your failures and don't make excuses. We don't need or want excuses."

Dillon speaks from experience. When he was nineteen, he sought out his biological parents. Again he met his mom at a park. While many things in her life had not changed, his mother accepted responsibility for what she did and wanted forgiveness and reconciliation. That was healing, and Dillon is hopeful there can be a new chapter for them. He also met with his father. Though his father showed no remorse, Dillon made peace with himself for having tried to repair the relationship. Through it all, he was grateful that he had his adoptive parents for support.

By most people's standards, Dillon's early life was difficult. When asked what he thinks about the argument that abortion spares kids from facing adversity, he says he gets where people are coming from. There were times when he was young, dealing with the pain of physical, sexual, and emotional abuse, that he had wished he had never been born.

But…through his tears, he says he is so glad that the desire of his early years to have never been born wasn't realized and that his birth mom made the choice she did to give him life. If he had never been born, he wouldn't now be newly married to the woman of his dreams, with the hopes of starting a family of his own. Although he experienced pain and suffering, Dillon feels God had mercy upon him, and he is walking more in His light every day. Now he can be a voice to those in similar situations and bring light to their darkness.

"Life can be really, really hard. But dream big and don't let go of that dream. Because to the extent life has been bad, it can be that good too," he says before planting a kiss on the cheek of his bride, who also happens to be my daughter Jazzi.

Chapter 10

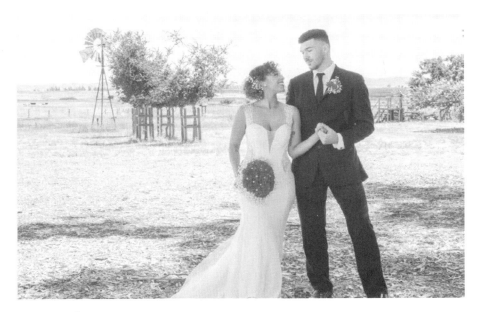

Jazzi & Dillon
Photography by SuzetteAllen.com

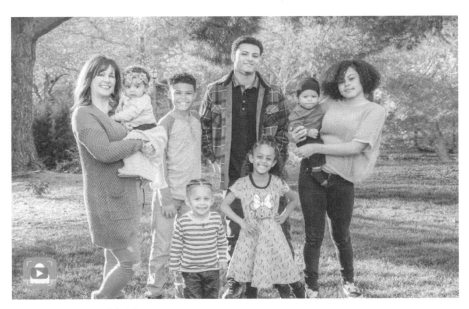

Laura & her grandchildren
Photography by SuzetteAllen.com

CHAPTER 11

It Isn't Finished

So there you have it: my story and some of the stories of those whom I love—all flawed, all made beautiful by God's amazing grace. They are solid proof that nothing can separate us from the love of God.

The stories in these pages have their fair share of the kinds of trauma and injustice that could leave a person reeling. I mean, who would blame a victim of abuse and sex-trafficking for making the rounds and just surviving? Not me. But I am inspired that so many have chosen to do more than just survive. They have chosen zoe.

We aren't defined by our past. My sister Barb passed down a profound truth to me: Looking at your past can lead to depression, looking ahead to anxiety, but being in the moment is truly living. The stains of sin and shame, trauma and poor choices, they are not permanent. The wages of sin *is* death, but...

BUT...the gift of God is eternal life. Jesus scorned shame, and His spirit inside us gives us the power to do likewise. He took the keys to death and unlocked eternal life for us. We were created to live the zoe

life, and He is hovering over our chaos, bringing order and beauty…
and *life*.

Deuteronomy 30:19 NIV says, "This day I call the heavens and
the earth as witnesses against you that I have set before you life and
death, blessings and curses. Now choose life, so that you and your
children may live."

Showing mercy and compassion, sacrificing for others, choosing
hope in the face of despair, and believing we serve a good God who
has our future in His hands—that's what living the zoe life is all
about. Bringing others to live under this truth, to take part of the
Tree of Zoe, that is our purpose. It is time to lead by speaking truth,
always in love.

When we choose zoe, we offer hope, and when we offer hope, we
save lives.

We must take active steps, such as those suggested in this book,
to build healthy relationships with our kids, to help women facing
unplanned pregnancy or the possibility of a disabled child, those
considering abortion or trying to heal from it, and those struggling
with miscarriage, infertility, or adoption. Further, we must find
ways to show regard for all life. We can guide children and church
members in making sacrifices of time and money for ministries that
care for the marginalized—the unborn, homeless, infirm, elderly,
disabled, imprisoned, or immigrant. We should promote and assist
organizations that help women in crisis pregnancy, donate blood,
befriend and include people who are differently abled and from
different ethnic and socio-economic backgrounds, provide safe
and welcoming worship environments for families dealing with

disabilities or socio-emotional issues, and read and discuss life-affirming books with our children.[75]

When it comes to challenging abortion specifically, here are some options:

- **Seek education** on abortion. Facts change the way people think.
- **Engage** with other pro-life people.
- **Inspire** the next generation to be pro-life.
- **Spearhead** a ministry at your church.
- **Volunteer** at your local pregnancy center.
- **Advocate** for life.
- **Pray** to end abortion.
- **Participate** in the *40 Days for Life* campaign.
- **Walk** in a yearly *Walk for Life*.
- **Donate** to pro-life organizations and pregnancy centers.
- **Offer hope**—evangelism begins in the womb.
- **Attend** pro-life banquets and keep up with pro-life events.
- **Share** your experience with people in a loving way. Testimonies are powerful. Social media can be vital in changing attitudes.
- **Be the change** by using your own gifts, writing, photography, and art, or by counselling and mentoring.
- **Show** your own ultrasounds. Images change the way people feel about abortion.
- **Teach** about fetal development. Equip yourself, family, and others with this information.
- **Research** and support pro-life candidates.
- **Work** to pass pro-life laws or even run for office.

- **Help** single mothers in your circle. Change two lives through compassion and kindness.
- **Know** what the Bible says about life, and carry that kingdom culture to the world.
- **Love**. Pure and simple, *love* is the answer to change hearts.

My personal struggles, joys, and choices have helped me to encourage others to choose life in the womb and a full life beyond, but my passion for choosing zoe didn't start with me. I was gifted with a rich family tradition of it. Charity sets the climate for generations to choose life, unmoved by situations that change as weather patterns do.

If you will, bear with me for one last story.

One summer day in the late 1920s, the "big sky" over the Augusta, Montana, farmland was weighed down with black, ominous clouds. Though still a young married couple, my grandparents and their five stairstep children were already entrenched in their community. That day, my grandpa kept an uneasy eye on the sky. Their vast wheat crop was nearing maturity, and their livelihood for the coming year was riding on its successful harvest. He turned toward the house, eager to share his concern with my grandma, but then remembered she wasn't there. "Nurse" was one of the many hats she wore, and she had been called away to town to help deliver a baby. He nervously went inside to check on the children.

It wasn't long before a loud clap of thunder and a cacophony of pounding brought him outside. He and his neighbors raced to secure the farm animals and then attempted to protect the wheat. It was futile. In the end, they sat helplessly under the protection of the roof as softball-sized hail beat his beautiful wheat crop into the ground.

Meanwhile, my grandma was bringing new life into the world. She knew what this storm would mean to them, but she tried to block out those thoughts and focus on the task at hand. The delivery went smoothly, and as my grandma prepared to leave, she steeled herself for the destruction and despair she would find when she arrived back on the farm.

From a distance, she could see that the wheat crop was indeed gone, and her heart sank. But though she found the destruction she expected, she did not find the despair. Instead, what she found was my grandpa shoveling the hail and making ice cream for the children and financially ruined neighbors. That day, and in the days to come, he chose and offered hope over despair. He sacrificed his resources to help others. He believed God had a bright future for his family in spite of a dismal present.

He chose zoe. And he helped his neighbors do the same. The world is counting on us to choose zoe and offer hope, just as my grandpa did. A child may enter the world amidst a storm, but that does not remove the chance for a sweet future.

Choosing an abundant life in the midst of pain, sorrow, and heartache may seem daunting, but start with the "one." It just takes giving to *one* person. Surely it is by giving that we receive what we need in return, and that is the essence of "choosing zoe." Choosing zoe has a way of snowballing. God only asks us to be faithful, and He will bring the increase. We will never bless others if we wait until all our ducks are in a row, our needs are met, or our lives are perfect. God does not require perfection. He is the master of bringing beauty out of ashes, of calmly hovering over the chaotic waters of our situation and bringing order. My life, and the lives of the other beautiful people who have graced the pages of this book, is proof of just that. These featured people represent all of us. They took their vulnerability and turned it into courage so others may behold life.

Jesus was born under chaotic circumstances. It doesn't get much messier than an animal shelter in a country under oppressive occupation, born in what the world perceived as a shotgun wedding. Yet Christ remains the perfect embodiment of zoe. Could it be that our heavenly Father is showing us that the circumstances surrounding birth do not define value or future? Perhaps He wants mothers to know that bringing forth life, regardless of situation, can have a profound reward? Or is He calling the church to rise up and be a beacon of hope to women who have not had the good fortune of being visited and comforted by an angel? Are *we* to be God's angels of mercy?

Yes, yes, and yes!

We have found beauty in chaos for a reason. We were introduced to the zoe life for a purpose. There is room under the Tree of Zoe for others. We are to be the voice of compassion to the woman who is plagued with guilt over her abortion and to the one who thinks keeping an unplanned pregnancy means her life is over.

No, it isn't over.

It's just the beginning.

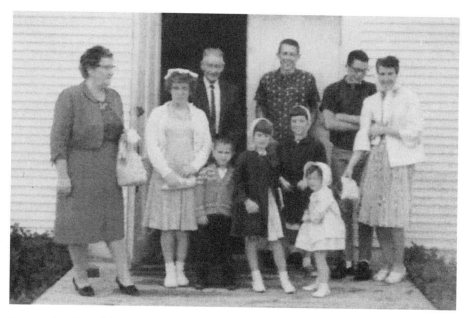

Laura's family with her grandparents, John & Vern Manix

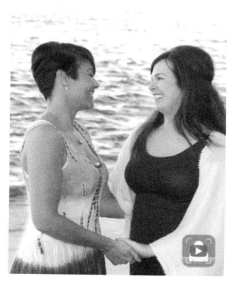

Laura & Arica at age 40
Capitola Beach

1. Tiffany Cheung, via written email correspondence with the author, April 20, 2017.

2. "Planned Parenthood Annual Report 2014-2015," *Planned Parenthood*, p. 28, accessed February 20, 2017, https://www. plannedparenthood.org/files/2114/5089/0863/2014-2015_ PPFA_Annual_Report_.pdf. See 4 above, page 30.

3. "Welcome to Alpha Pregnancy Clinics of Northern California," *Alpha Pregnancy Clinics*, accessed June 8, 2017, http://www.alphaclinics.org/about-us/welcome.

4. "How do I get the abortion pill?," *Planned Parenthood*, accessed February 20, 2017, https://www.plannedparenthood. org/learn/abortion/the-abortion-pill/how-do-i-get-the-abortion-pill?gclid=CLeW_PaRrNMCFQt_fgodB9sIVQ.

5. http://abortionworker.com/.

6. Beth Jones, Interview with Vanessa Chandler, March 15, 2017.

7. Barry and Lori Byrne, interview with Vanessa Chandler, February 1, 2017.

8. A sexual education ministry of Alpha Care Center, http:// alpha-pregnancycenter.org/.

9. Byrne.

10. Bill Muehlenberg, "Daughters and Dads Fact Sheet," *Dads4Kids.org*, August 2014, http://www.dads4kids.org.au/ resources/DADS-AND-DAUGHTERS.pdf.

11. Muehlenberg, and Carl E. Pickhardt, Ph.D., "Adolescence and Physical Affection with Parents," *Psychology Today*, November 26, 2012, https://www.psychologytoday.com/blog/

surviving-your-childs-adolescence/201211/adolescence-and-physical-affection-parents.

12. Alison Gee, "A world without Down's syndrome?," *BBC News Magazine*, September 29, 2016, http://www.bbc.com/news/magazine-37500189.

13. Susan Donaldson James, "Down Syndrome Births Are Down in U.S.," *ABC News*, November 2, 2009, http://abcnews.go.com/Health/w_ParentingResource/down-syndrome-births-drop-us-women-abort/story?id=8960803.

14. Hayley Goleniowska, "The Disability Abortion Lie," *The Huffington Post*, last modified November 25, 2014, http://www.huffingtonpost.co.uk/hayley-goleniowska/abortion-and-disability_b_5881256.html.

15. "Appeal to the United Nations," *Downpride.com*, November 9, 2015, https://downpride.com/appeal-to-the-united-nations/.

16. Gee.

17. Gee, and "Appeal to the United Nations."

18. James.

19. David Wasserman and Adrienne Asch, "The Uncertain Rationale for Prenatal Disability Screening," *AMA Journal of Ethics 8*, no. 1 (2006): 53-56, accessed February 20, 2017, http://journalofethics.ama-assn.org/2006/01/oped2-0601.html.

20. Goleniowska.

21. Beth Daley, "Oversold and misunderstood: Prenatal screening tests prompt abortions," *The Eye, from the New England Center for Investigative Reporting*, December 13, 2014, https://eye.necir.org/2014/12/13/prenatal-testing/.

22. Gee.

23. Psalm 139:13-14, 16 New International Version

24. Margaret Sanger and Carrie Chapman Catt, *The Pivot of Civilization* (New York: Bretano's, 1922), accessed February 8, 2017, http://groups.csail.mit.edu/mac/users/rauch/abortion_eugenics/sanger/sanger_04.html.

25. Margaret Sanger, *Woman and the New Race*, (New York: Bretano's, 1920), accessed February 20, 2017, http://www.bartleby.com/1013/18.html.

26. "The Genocide of Mental Disability: An examination of the fine line between preventative medicine and genocidal eugenics," *Northern Michigan University*, accessed March 7, 2017, http://www.nmu.edu/english/sites/DrupalEnglish/files/UserFiles/WritingAwards/Cohodas/Genocide_of_Mental_Disability.pdf.

27. Goleniowska.

28. "PPFA Annual Report 2014-2015," *Planned Parenthood*, 32, accessed February 9, 2017, https://www.plannedparenthood.org/files/2114/5089/0863/2014-2015_PPFA_Annual_Report_.pdf.

29. Championsclub.org.

30. Tim Tebow Foundation, http://www.timtebowfoundation.org/index.php/night-to-shine/

31. Peter Nieman and Sarah Shea, "Effective Discipline for Children," *The U.S. National Institutes of Health's National Library of Medicine 9*, no.1 (2004): 37-41, accessed March 7, 2017, https://www.ncbi.nlm.nih.gov/pmc/articles/PMC2719514/.

32. "House Resolution No. 214," *Virginia's Legislative Information System*, January 23, 1015, accessed May 30, 2017, https://lis. virginia.gov/cgi-bin/legp604.exe?151+ful+HR214.

33. "Planned Parenthood Annual Report 2014-2015," *Planned Parenthood*, p. 10, accessed February 20, 2017, https://www. plannedparenthood.org/files/2114/5089/0863/2014-2015_ PPFA_Annual_Report_.pdf.

34. G. Donald Royster, interview by Jennifer Bell, March 23, 2017.

35. "Prenatal Summary," *The Endowment for Human Development*, accessed March 10, 2017, https://www.ehd.org/prenatal-summary.php.

36. "Hearing Before the Subcommittee on the Constitution and Civil Justice on H.R 1797, District of Columbia Pain-Capable Unborn Child Protection Act," *Committee on the Judiciary House of Representatives*, May 23, 2013, p. 36-46, https:// www.gpo.gov/fdsys/pkg/CHRG-113hhrg81175/pdf/CHRG-113hhrg81175.pdf.

37. "Derrick's Story – Faces of Life Contest 3rd Place," *Focus on the Family* via *YouTube*, November 9, 2011, https://www.youtube. com/watch?v=ROn5GzQ4AYE&list=PLN_OwL4J8L1B4cPEQ-WsHYP8uD4I5Mli-&index=3.

38. CB, Interview with Vanessa Chandler, March 28, 2017.

39. "N.T. Wright on What It Means to Be An Image Bearer," *The Biologos Foundation*, June 16, 2010, accessed May 30, 2017, https://www.youtube.com/watch?v=yp-Ku-_ekAY.

40. Christine Caine, *Unashamed*, p.43, Zondervan Publishing, March 2016.

41. "CDCs Abortion Surveillance System FAQs," *Centers for Disease Control and Prevention*, updated January 6, 2016, https://www.cdc.gov/reproductivehealth/data_stats/abortion.htm.

42. Michelle Ye Hee Lee, "The stale claim that 'one in three' women will have an abortion by the age of 45," *The Washington Post*, September 30, 2015, https://www.washingtonpost.com/news/fact-checker/wp/2015/09/30/the-stale-claim-that-one-in-three-women-will-have-an-abortion-by-age-45/?utm_term=.317a6d9b680f.

43. Heather Wood Rudulph, "Why I Filmed My Abortion," *Cosmopolitan*, May 5, 2014, http://www.cosmopolitan.com/politics/a6674/why-i-filmed-my-abortion/.

44. Whitney Bell, "What to Get a Friend Post-Abortion," *TeenVogue*, January 20, 2017, http://www.teenvogue.com/gallery/post-abortion-gift-guide.

45. "Parental Consent and Notification Laws," *Planned Parenthood*, accessed April 18, 2017, https://www.plannedparenthood.org/learn/abortion/parental-consent-notification-laws.

46. Valerie Richardson, "Colorado abortion clinic staff failed to report 13-yr-old's sexual abuse," *The Washington Times*, July 29, 2015, http://www.washingtontimes.com/news/2015/jul/29/planned-parenthood-failed-to-report-13-year-old-gi/., Natalie Decker, "Planned Parenthood's 'Don't Ask, Don't Tell' Policy Victimizes Children," *The Gazette*, May 31, 2015, http://gazette.com/guest-column-planned-parenthoods-dont-ask-dont-tell-policy-victimizes-children/article/1552840.

47. "Planned Parenthood Annual Report 2014-2015," *Planned Parenthood*, p. 28, accessed February 20, 2017, https://www.plannedparenthood.org/files/2114/5089/0863/2014-2015_PPFA_Annual_Report_.pdf.

48. Michelle Ye Hee Lee, "For Planned Parenthood abortion stats, '3 percent' and '94 percent' are both misleading," *The Washington Post*, August 12, 2015, https://www.washingtonpost.com/news/fact-checker/wp/2015/08/12/for-planned-parenthood-abortion-stats-3-percent-and-94-percent-are-both-misleading/?utm_term=.ca6ba6e30b37.

49. Based upon most recent data available at the time of writing.

50. "Planned Parenthood Annual Report 2014-2015," page 30.

51. Georgette Forney, "The Reality of Abortion," Silent No More, August 11, 2008, http://www.silentnomoreawareness.org/articles/article.aspx?articleid=91&owner=0.

52. G. Donald Royster, interview by Jennifer Bell, March 23, 2017.

53. "Written Testimony of Kathi A. Aultman, MD, Senate Judiciary Committee Hearing March 15, 2016," *U.S. Senate,* https://www.judiciary.senate.gov/imo/media/doc/03-15-16%20Aultman%20Testimony.pdf.

54. Doe v. Bolton. 70-40. United States Supreme Court. 1973. Accessed April 10, 2017, http://caselaw.findlaw.com/us-supreme-court/410/179.html.

55. Serena, in discussion with the author, April 2017.

56. Georgette Forney, interview by Jennifer Bell, February 11, 2017.

57. Lesley Samuels, in discussion with the author, April 28, 2017.

58. Susanne Babbel, "Post Abortion Stress Syndrome (PASS) –

Does it Exist?", *Psychology Today*, October 25, 2010, https://www.psychologytoday.com/blog/somatic-psychology/201010/post-abortion-stress-syndrome-pass-does-it-exist.

59. Babbel.

60. Georgette Forney, "The Reality of Abortion," Silent No More, August 11, 2008, http://www.silentnomoreawareness.org/articles/article.aspx?articleid=91&owner=0.

61. Grazie Pozo Christie, "Let's Compare Studies to See if Abortion Really Harms Women's Mental Health," *The Federalist*, April 24, 2017, https://thefederalist.com/2017/04/24/lets-compare-studies-see-abortion-really-harms-womens-mental-health/.

62. Georgette Forney, interview by Jennifer Bell, February 11, 2017.

63. Arica Henry Ports, interview with Vanessa Chandler, December 19, 2016.

64. Ben Folds Five, "Brick," *Whatever and Ever Amen*, Epic, November 21, 1997.

65. Forney interview.

66. G. Donald Royster, interview with Jennifer Bell, March 23, 2017.

67. Janice, interview with Jennifer Bell, January 29, 2017.

68. Dillon Milton, interview with the author, March 13, 2017.

69. "How Many Couples are Waiting to Adopt?," *American Adoption*, accessed March 27, 2017, http://www.americanadoptions.com/pregnant/article_view/article_id/4517?cId=149.

70. Courtney Jacobson, interview with Jennifer Bell, March 20, 2017.

71. Janice, interview with Jennifer Bell, January 29, 2017.

72. Survey conducted March 14, 2017.

73. Sophia Cruz, interview with Jennifer Bell, March 20, 2017.

74. Ephesians 1:3-5 English Standard Version.

75. "5 Pro-Life Picture Books Your Kids Will Love," *American Life League's Culture of Life Studies Program*, October 6, 2016, http://cultureoflifestudies.com/blog/5-pro-life-picture-books-your-kids-will-love/.

Appendix A

Abortion – Dangers

1. Silent No More's "What's So Bad About Abortion?"
    Download or order here:
    http://www.silentnomoreawareness.org/articles/article.
    aspx?articleid=85&owner=0

2. Anglicans for Life's "Women's Health: Abortion"
    Download or order here:
    https://vps33368.inmotionhosting.com/~anglicansforlife/
    archive/womens-health-and-abortion/

3. Family Research Council's "Planned Parenthood: What Every
    Parent, Teacher, Woman, Community Leader and Elected
    Official Needs to Know"
    Download here: http://downloads.frc.org/EF/EF10I10.pdf

Abortions – Forced

1. The center against forced abortion: thejusticefoundation.org/cafa/

Abortion – Healing

1. A Movement of Love: www.amovementoflove.org
2. Rachel's Vineyard: Rachelsvineyard.org
3. Abortion Recovery Network: www.abortionrecovery.org
   National hotline: 657-464-7071
4. International helpline for abortion recovery: www.internationalhelpline.org
   National toll-free hotline: 1-866-482-LIFE (1-866-482-5433)
5. Elliot Institute: Afterabortion.org
6. Priests for Life: Priestsforlife.org
7. Abort 73—Unfiltered stories of women and men who have experienced the painful aftermath of abortion: www.abort73.com
8. The Silent No More Awareness Campaign: www.silentnomoreawareness.org

Abortion – Healing for Men

1. The UnChoice: theunchoice.com
2. Healing Tears: healingtears.org/healing-men-and-abortion/

Abortion – Minors

1. Parental consent and notification laws for abortion by minors–
   state requirements:
   www.plannedparenthood.org/learn/abortion/parental-
   consent-notification-laws

Adoption

1. Bethany Christian Services, adoption assistance: www.bethany.
   org
2. Karyn Purvis, David Cross, and Wendy Sunshine, *The Connected Child: Bring Hope and Healing to Your Adopted Family* (New York: McGraw-Hill, 2007)
3. Focus on the Family: www.focusonthefamily.com/pro-life/
   orphan-care

Disabilities – Creating Support and a Place to Thrive

1. The Champions Club: championsclub.org
2. Mikey's Place: mikeysplace.net
3. Focus on the Family: focusonthefamily.com, Option Ultrasound

Kids – Creating a Culture of Life

1. "5 Pro-Life Picture Books Your Kids Will Love," *American Life*

League's Culture of Life Studies Program, October 6, 2016
http://cultureoflifestudies.com/blog/5-pro-life-picture-books-your-kids-will-love/

Miscarriage and Pregnancy Loss

1. Kathe Wunnenberg, *Grieving the Child I Never Knew* (Grand Rapids, MI: Zondervan, 2001)
2. Gwen Kik and Teale Fackler, *Threads of Hope, Pieces of Joy: A Pregnancy Loss Bible Study* (Benjamin Books, 1999)
3. Focus on the Family: www.focusonthefamily.com/pro-life/preborn/pregnancy-and-infant-loss/pregnancy-and-infant-loss
4. Now I Lay Me Down To Sleep: www.nowilaymedowntosleep.org

Relationship Help

1. Nothing Hidden Ministries app developed by Barry Byrne— Toolkit to help those striving to make godly choices in relationships and singleness. Available from the app store for $2.99

Unplanned Pregnancy – Support

1. Alpha Pregnancy Clinics: www.alphaclinics.org
2. Heartbeat International: heartbeatinternational.org
3. Option Line: optionline.org, or text "HELPLINE" to 313131

4. YourOptions: www.youroptions.com

5. Real Options Medical Clinics: Realoptions.net

6. Care Net: www.care-net.org, Life Disciples Program Helpline: 877-791-5475

7. The Nurturing Network: nurturingnetwork.org/referral_resources_1/pregnancy_resources

8. Heidi Murkoff and Sharon Mazel, *What to Expect When You're Expecting* (New York: Workman Publishing Company, Inc., 2002)

9. Carey Wickersham, *The Wonder Within You: Celebrating Your Baby's Journey from Conception to Birth* (Carol Stream, IL: Tyndale House Publishers, 2014)

How the Church Can Help Women Heal from Abortion

Step 1: Develop a Team

Church leadership should begin by developing a team of both women and men who are passionate about helping others heal from abortion through serving as leaders for a ten-week healing process. Team members should attend post-abortive trainings and grief seminars, as well as pray continually for new insights to reach those affected by abortion. The hope is that people will experience healing and in turn be trained to lead their own healing.

Step 2: Develop Effective Outreach Using Existing Ministries

Church ministries, such as recovery programs, counseling, and in-depth, team-led prayer sessions, may present opportunities for post-abortive healing and recovery for those who have participated in abortion. Educate ministry leaders to encourage people who are suffering from abortion to come forward for help with healing.

Step 3: Demonstrate Compassionate Church Awareness

As scary as it may seem, church leadership needs to be bold in addressing the topic of abortion and the need for post-abortive healing. Simply ignoring it will not make it go away; it will just fester. Because some women were coerced into abortion by the men in their lives, and thus it is helpful to have a female pastor or a spiritually mature woman involved in presenting this topic.

When my pastors started their post-abortion healing ministry, A Movement of Love, they spoke together as senior pastors to the entire congregation, educating us regarding the scientific and spiritual facts about life beginning at the moment of conception. They compassionately helped our congregation understand that abortion is not God's will and He will forgive and heal those who have had them or partnered with them. They offered a support system to facilitate the healing process confidentially in a safe place.

In the five years A Movement of Love has existed, we have used different ways to touch on the subject of abortion:

- Education on Life Sunday—Highlighting concrete scientific facts of the developing baby in the womb.
- Sermons—Taking a biblical perspective on ideas such as, "if it's

legal, it's okay," and emphasizing that legalizing abortion does not make the moral dilemma go away.

- Skits—Presenting a three-part skit called "Unthinkable" during the Sunday sermon, which portrays three stories of crisis pregnancy, abortion, and redemption after the abortion.
- Men's voices—Inviting guest male speakers to share their testimonies of abortion and forgiveness to the men's ministry group.
- Informational nights—Inviting women through the weekly event video to an informational night where they can hear from women who have gone through the healing process share their stories. Attendees are encouraged to go through the process themselves. Interactives work well during the information night, as women realize they can be heard and healed in the context of community.
- Videos—Posting videos on the church website that discuss abortion's effect on women and the opportunity to receive healing. The videos cover various topics and include testimonies from women who have gone through the healing process.

Step 4: Provide a Place to Heal

Church leaders should prayerfully consider adopting a study specifically designed for healing from abortion. My church offers a ten-week study called *Forgiven and Set Free* by Linda Cochrane, and there are several other quality resources available as well.

This is obviously a sensitive topic for people. Discretion and confidentiality are a must. Connecting people to the group leader or a facilitator is a way to help those who express interest in joining.

At our church, once a woman decides that she is indeed interested, she completes a confidential intake form, which is followed up by an interview. The purpose of the interview is to ensure that she is ready to go through the healing process and can commit to the entire ten to twelve weeks. Often, this is the first time a woman is able to confide the secret of her abortion. Less than two weeks transpire between the informational meeting and the beginning of the study.

Once the study begins, each participant signs a confidentiality agreement and a commitment for regular attendance. The meetings take place discreetly in a ministry room of the church, just like a Bible study or other ministry gathering. They last for ninety minutes, and childcare is provided. Many pregnancy centers offer these studies, but I find it powerful restorative justice when churches offer them.

Information graciously provided by Joan West, founder of A Movement of Love and pastor at Liberty Church in Fairfield, California.

Ideas for Effecting Change Regarding Abortion

Seek education on abortion. Facts change the way people think.

Engage with other pro-life people.

Inspire the next generation to be pro-life.

Spearhead a ministry at your church.

Volunteer at your local pregnancy center.

Advocate for life.

Pray to end abortion.

Participate in the *40 Days for Life* campaign.

Walk in a yearly *Walk for Life*.

Donate to pro-life organizations and pregnancy centers.

Offer hope—evangelism begins in the womb.

Attend pro-life banquets and keep up with pro-life events.

Share your experience with people in a loving way. Testimonies are powerful. Social media can be vital in changing attitudes.

Be the change by using your own gifts, writing, photography, and art, or by counseling and mentoring.

Show your own ultrasounds. Images change the way people feel about abortion.

Teach about fetal development. Equip yourself, family, and others with this information.

Research and support pro-life candidates.

Work to pass pro-life laws or even run for office.

Help single mothers in your circle. Change two lives through compassion and kindness.

Know what the Bible says about life, and carry that kingdom culture to the world.

Love. Pure and simple, *love* is the answer to change hearts.

ACKNOWLEDGEMENTS

Conception

Dear God,

Thank you for sharing your heartbeat for your created ones. I cried out to you on behalf of pregnant teens, and you heard my cry. As a first-time author, you trusted me and gave me vision to deliver the message of Zoe.

You gave me grandparents oozing with love and civility, and parents who embody the culture of life. Dad instilled the Imagio Dei mantra, Momma impressed how love begins with family, and my siblings continue to encourage me with endless support and cheer me on.

You graced me with five children. My legacy of love—Arica, Geoffrey, Amanda, Jazzi and Mary who blessed me with son-in-loves, plus the joys of my life: eight grandchildren thus far.

> *"Behold children are a heritage from the Lord, the fruit of the womb a reward (Psalm 127:3)."*

Development

Alpha Pregnancy Clinic: You gave me a platform to advocate for life. Together we have co-labored following generations of pro-life heroes to save children, and their parents. I can confidently proclaim, "We are winning!"

Choose Zoe

My Liberty Church family, Pastors, and my small group:
Relationships with you has given me courage and empowered me
to thrive. It is such a pleasure to minister side-by-side and to do life
together. You've helped me through some of my most painful times,
and I'm forever grateful for your love and prayers.

Yes, it takes a village to raise a child, but friends make life worth
living. Friends who walk hand in hand, type my sticky notes, secure
and design websites, take photographs, help me market and listen
to all my crazy ideas. We dream together, weep and rejoice. Please
accept my heartfelt thankfulness for your devotion, innovation and
creativity.

Red Arrow Media: Your team grasped my vision. I felt so
enlivened when you understood my Zoe mission. Vanessa—You
coached me through the process with your gracious professional
care and edited my work. Jen Bell: When this novice writer couldn't
articulate, as some subjects were just too personal, your writing
gave me literary excellence. At times it felt like you were a surrogate
mother. With God we birthed *Choose Zoe* out of the darkness into the
glorious light.

Delivery

Thank you, God, for all the courageous people who shared
intimate stories of struggle and hope. My beloved children I carried,
whose love has equally carried me, laboring in love, making sure
I would not miscarry my dream. When I was screaming for an
epidural, you God gave me the miracle of life. I faced opposition, and
you gave supernatural strength to push through. Just like every child

born is a miracle, it is a true miracle that *Choose Zoe* is born.

"When a woman is giving birth, she has sorrow because her hour has come, but when she has delivered the baby, she no longer remembers the anguish, for joy that a human being has been born into the world" (John 16:21).

God, family was your idea and you love us all with an everlasting love. This book you entrusted me with is my offering to you, a labor of love and I hope you like it. I pray these words ignite hope and inspire all to choose life and choose you. I give you all glory and honor by living the abundant "zoe" life that your son Jesus came to give.

Your daughter, Laura

Option Line: Optionline.org or Text "HELPLINE" to 313131

Consultants are available in the US and Canada, 24 hours a day, 365 days a year, answering in both English and Spanish. Consultants answer questions by phone, text, email, or chat before connecting each woman with her local pregnancy help organization where she'll receive one-on-one compassionate, caring support.